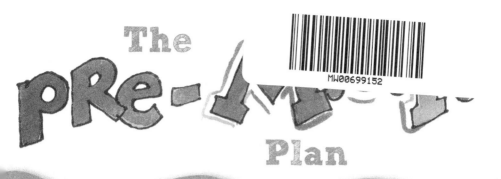

The PRe-M-O-P Plan

How to resolve constipation in babies and toddlers and overcome potty-training struggles

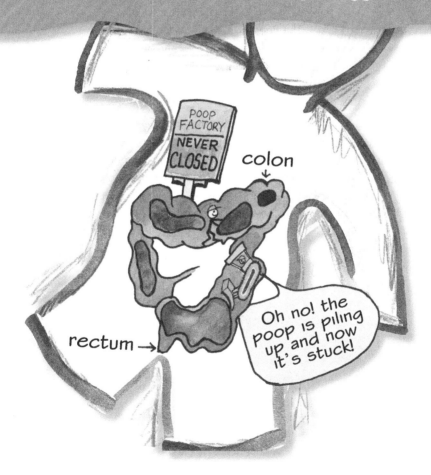

By Steve Hodges, M.D.
with Suzanne Schlosberg
Illustrated by Cristina Acosta

The Pre-M.O.P. Plan, 1st Edition
Text Copyright © 2019 Steve J. Hodges and Suzanne Schlosberg
Illustration Copyright © 2017 Cristina Acosta
Book design: DyanRothDesign.com

O'Regan press

Library of Congress Cataloging-in-Publication Data is available on file.

ISBN: 978-0-9908774-8-6

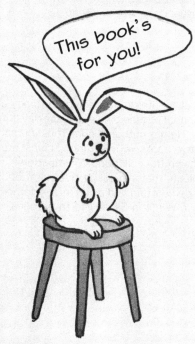

This book is dedicated to parents who've been told that "more fiber and prune juice" will do the job.

About the Authors

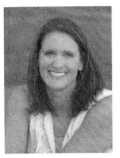

Suzanne Schlosberg

Suzanne is a health writer who specializes in translating clinical mumbo jumbo into English. Years ago, on a mission to achieve a diaper-free household. Suzanne potty-trained her twin boys too early; she used Steve Hodges' methods to undo the damage. The author or co-author of 20 books. Suzanne co-founded BedwettingAndAccidents.com with Dr. Hodges and manages the website. Her website is SuzanneSchlosbergWrites.com. Suzanne lives with her husband and boys in Bend. Oregon.

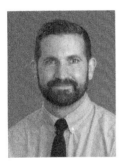

Steve Hodges, M.D.

Steve Hodges is an associate professor of pediatric urology at Wake Forest University School of Medicine and a specialist in childhood toileting issues. He has authored numerous journal articles and co-authored five books with Suzanne Schlosberg. His mission is to shed light on the childhood constipation epidemic and to communicate that aggressive treatment of constipation can prevent bedwetting and accidents. A father of three, Dr. Hodges lives in Winston-Salem. North Carolina.

About the Artist

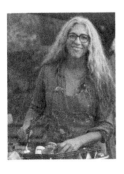

Cristina Acosta

Cristina is an artist who loves illustrating poop books.Though Cristina's daughter is long past potty training. Cristina is excited to help children grow up healthy and confident. When she's not visualizing the gastrointestinal tract. Cristina paints, draws and designs most anything she can. She divides her time between the Pacific Northwest and Southern California. Her website is CristinaAcosta.com.

Praise for
The pRe-M.O.P. Plan
From Medical Doctors!

"Mandatory reading for all pediatric care providers! Wonderfully, the anatomy, physiology, and science are delivered with a humorist's tone that invites smiles and relief about a topic that's usually embarrassing."
— Rob Paynter, M.D.
Pediatrician
Novant Health Forsyth Pediatrics
Winston Salem, North Carolina

"A book that will change lives! I urge parents, pediatricians, and specialists alike to take seriously Dr. Hodges' approach. So many of the problems I treat could be prevented by Pre-M.O.P."
— Irina Stanasel, M.D.
Pediatric Urologist,
UT Southwestern Medical Center
Dallas, Texas

"I sincerely thank Dr. Hodges for getting this message out. I hope the implementation of the plan in babies and toddlers will prevent years of suffering for school-age children and their families."
— James Sander, M.D.
Chief, Division of Urology
University of Texas Rio Grande Valley School of Medicine

"Concise and well-reasoned — and balanced with humor and wisdom. The recommendations are practical and specific while offering multiple options. This book will make potty training easier for both parent and child!"
— Michael Garrett, M.D.
Family physician and owner, Direct MD
Austin, Texas

"A wonderful resource for families and clinicians! This creative book recognizes the important relationship between the colon and the urinary system: Poor emptying of one can affect the emptying of the other, which can in turn have significant clinical and social implications.
— Marc A. Levitt, M.D.
Chief, Colorectal and Pelvic Reconstructive Surgery
Children's National Hospital
Washington D.C.

Table of Contents

Introduction

What My Patients and Your Child Have in Common

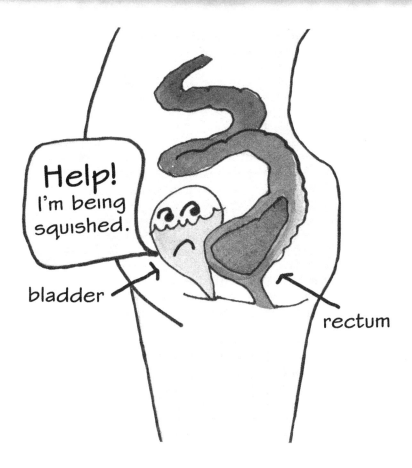

"I took him to the ER when he hadn't had a poop in over a week. An x-ray showed enormous constipation, but the doctor simply suggested Miralax. Miralax did nothing."

My clinic at Wake Forest University is filled with children of all ages — 4-year-olds, 5th-graders, teenagers — who struggle with bedwetting, daytime pee accidents, or poop accidents. Or in many cases, all three.

Most of these kids were assured by their doctors, year after year, that accidents are normal.

"Don't worry," their doctors would say. "You'll outgrow it."

But these kids didn't, and now the accidents are causing them and their families immense distress.

As the mom of a 5-year-old with poop accidents (encopresis) described it:

> *We can't plan a trip, and we can't get a sitter, because he will just poop, sit in it, and not tell anyone. He's immune to the smell of it and doesn't realize he's doing it. I have to change his pants literally 5 times a day. He's starting big school in September and I'm so terrified that he will be picked on.*

Her fear is warranted. Many of my patients are teased, even bullied, at school. ("This kid poops his pants!" "He stinks!") Some have been suspended or threatened with suspension. Some are homeschooled because their accidents have become unmanageable. Many of these kids miss out on birthday sleepovers and school trips. A few have had to defer admission to college because, well, no one wants to bring giant pull-ups to their dorm room.

I know these scenarios do not describe your child. Your child is just a baby or a toddler, maybe a young preschooler, and all this probably sounds like someone else's nightmare.

But my patients and your child have something in common: chronic constipation.

Your baby's pooping trouble is the precursor to the accidents that plague my school-age patients.

How so?

Well, when children delay pooping, as they often do, stool piles up in the rectum, which is a stretchy and accommodating organ, though not one designed as a storage facility. Over time — months, years — a stool-stuffed rectum can stretch to two or three times its normal diameter. But a child's body, with numerous organs packed into a small space, does not have room for a super-sized rectum. It's crowded in there!

So, the rectum starts to press against the nearby bladder. At the same time, the enlarged rectum stretches and aggravates the nerves that control bladder emptying, triggering the bladder to empty without warning, day or night. That's what is happening when toilet-trained kids pee in their pants (enuresis) or wet the bed (nocturnal enuresis).

"Around 8 months I noticed poop pellets and straining but didn't see it as a huge problem until potty training at age 2, when she would hide and squat down to try to hold poop in until we gave her a diaper. She had poop accidents from potty training on. Our doctor only ever recommended pear juice as a baby, and we started Miralax at age 3. Looking back, I would have put potty training on hold from the moment she started hiding and withholding."

In some cases, the rectum becomes so stretched that it loses its tone, the way a stretched-out sock loses elasticity, and can't pump stool out the door with enough oomph. The floppy rectum loses sensation, too, so the child no longer feels the urge to poop. At that point, stool just drops out of the child's bottom, often without the child noticing. That's encopresis.

At the risk of sounding alarmist, I will be blunt: If you don't resolve your baby's constipation now — I mean, really, *really* resolve it — the condition is likely to worsen, and your child may end up with a chronically enlarged rectum. Eventually, your baby may become a 5th grader who leaves behind poop pellets on play dates, a 13-year-old who is too embarrassed to go on Boy Scout overnights, or a 10th-grader who packs nine garbage bags on a trip to Rome with the Latin club, hoping to keep his mattress dry. Those are three of my patients.

These patients, like virtually all the kids I see in clinic, became constipated well before age 3. Even in patients whose accidents didn't begin until kindergarten or later, the signs of constipation were evident early on, and they were missed.

My patients' constipation can invariably be traced back to one of three eras in their young lives:

1) **infancy**

2) **at the introduction of solid foods (between 4 and 12 months) or cow's milk (around 1 year)**

3) **during toilet training (between 18 months and 3 years)**

The parents who visit my clinic or who join our private Facebook support group wish they had recognized the red flags earlier. They wish they had treated their children's constipation more aggressively and followed up with more vigilance. They wish their doctors had done the same.

As one mom in our support group posted:

I wish I hadn't continued to believe "He'll grow out of it" when my gut told me something was off. But when you have an otherwise healthy baby, you NEVER think that the infant whose constipation your pediatrician deems "normal" could eventually turn into a 4 1/2-year-old who never poops on his own and gets an enema every night. In retrospect, I wish I had been all over the constipation when he was a baby. It's so frustrating to think, What if I had been more aggressive back then?

My goal is to save your family from this frustration.

By resolving your child's chronic constipation now — before withholding becomes a more deeply ingrained habit and before the rectum becomes persistently stretched — you may well save your child from years of discomfort, distress, and damaged self-esteem. You may also save yourself from 2 a.m. bedding changes and the expense of extra-large pull-ups, plus the financial and emotional costs of treating enuresis and encopresis.

It's critical to nip all this in the bud before your child enters the school system, because that's when the crap really hits the fan!

School restroom policies commonly and deliberately encourage withholding. Many schools dangle prizes for not using bathroom passes — students can earn trinkets, even pizza parties, for ignoring their bodies' signals. Some students must pay, in fake classroom currency, for the "privilege" of using the toilet. Even when kids are excused to use the restroom, they are often viewed with suspicion or rushed. As one mom posted, "At our school, the teachers stand at the bathroom door and yell at the kids to hurry up."

Not long ago, 1st-grade teachers in Las Vegas sent parents a letter stating that "students are wasting valuable learning time on bathroom breaks" and insisting 6-year-olds need only pee once or twice during the school day. The teachers asked parents to help their children "increase bladder endurance" by overriding their urges to pee. After a backlash from parents, the principal retracted the letter and conceded that unfettered restroom access is a "a basic human right and need." But clearly the school's teachers, like plenty of teachers elsewhere, misunderstand some basic facts about bladder health.

I have plenty of patients who never, ever use the toilet at school, because their schools restrict access or because they're too grossed out or afraid of being teased or bullied. This makes it even tougher for these students to overcome enuresis and encopresis. Holding pee thickens and irritates the bladder, exacerbating the symptoms caused by holding poop.

Believe me: Compared to resolving chronic constipation in a tween or teen, fixing the problem in a baby or toddler is easy!

This book is aimed at helping children who show signs of chronic constipation before they have toilet trained, as well as youngsters who are currently training and are struggling to poop on the potty.

Early Intervention is Everything

Many physicians dismiss constipation in babies and toddlers as a minor, temporary condition that can be resolved with prune juice and a more nutritious diet, plus maybe some fiber gummies and an occasional dose of laxative. Nothing to worry about here! She'll outgrow it!

One mom in our support group, whose son became constipated as a toddler, posted that she was unaware of the warning signs:

> *By the time he was 2 1/2, he had encopresis. I didn't know what it was, but I knew it wasn't normal. Our nurse practitioner suggested more fruits and vegetables in his diet, drinking prune juice, limiting dairy and processed foods. I drove myself to madness trying to restrict my son's diet, but the encopresis only got worse . . . to the point where he just stopped having bowel movements and only had skid marks in his diaper for 10 days. I took him to the ER when he hadn't had a poop in over a week. An x-ray showed enormous constipation, but the doctor simply suggested Miralax. Miralax did nothing.*

That's what the most commonly prescribed treatments do: nothing!

Research confirms the uselessness of common remedies. Despite treatment, only 50 to 70 percent of children with functional constipation demonstrate long-term improvement. University of Michigan physicians concluded.[1] In one study cited by the Michigan doctors, 52% of children with constipation and

---

1   Wendy S. Biggs and William Dery. "Evaluation and Treatment of Constipation in Infants and Children." *American Family Physician*, 1;73(3). Feb. 2006: 469-477. https://www.aafp.org/afp/2006/0201/p469.html.

encopresis still had symptoms after five years of treatment.[2]

That's a pretty lousy success rate!

"Functional" constipation, by the way, means constipation not caused by an underlying medical condition, such as a congenital abnormality or disease. Overall, at least 95% of constipation cases in children fall into the "functional" category, and in children over age 1, the percentage is higher — 99% in my practice. (I discuss the exceptions in Part 1.)

Now, just because treatment commonly fails and the relapse rate is high does not mean childhood constipation is an intractable condition. Not at all! It just means the common remedies are falling short. Way short. When you treat constipation with half measures, you shouldn't be surprised that only half of constipated kids, or fewer, will find relief.

"Aggressive" Treatment is the Only Treatment Worth Doing

I have described the risks of under-treating constipation in babies and explained that you can draw a straight line from constipation in infancy to bedwetting in high school. What I haven't yet described is the treatment required to fully, permanently resolve enuresis and encopresis.

That treatment is the Modified O'Regan Protocol, known as **M.O.P.**, and involves daily enemas. Yes, daily — as in *every single day*. Usually for months. In some cases, for over a year. Yes, that's a ton of enemas. Yes, it's safe. And yes, it's necessary.

By the time a child is constipated enough to have developed enuresis or encopresis, oral laxatives alone fall far short (though they play a helpful, secondary role in resolving these conditions). Laxatives soften stool, but the newer, mushier poop will just ooze around the mondo mountain blocking the tunnel. At that point, even blasting through the clog with a colonoscopy-grade laxative — what humorist Dave Barry once called a "nuclear"

2 A., Staiano, et al., "Long-term follow-up of children with chronic idiopathic constipation, *Digestive Diseases and Sciences*, 1994, 39:561–4, https://link.springer.com/article/10.1007/BF02088343.

> *"We started seeing pediatric GIs at 6 months. All three prescribed laxatives only — Miralax, Natural Calm, Dulcolax, senna. Nothing worked. At age 3, after potty training, she was diagnosed with encopresis. I read about M.O.P. and we started doing liquid glycerin suppositories every day, and that's when things started improving. Total lifesaver! We did LGS daily for 6 months. Then one day she said she wanted to poop on the potty, and she did!! Now we do LGS every once in a while, but for the most part, it's solved."*

laxative[3] — is a temporary fix, at best.

That's because cleaning out the rectum is only half the battle. The more important goal is giving the rectum a chance to shrink back to its normal size and regain tone and sensation. None of that will happen unless the rectum is fully evacuated every day for months. Since these kids are superstar withholders, and because large, hard mounds of stool don't disintegrate on contact with Miralax or milk of magnesia, more powerful measures are needed. Ergo: M.O.P.

M.O.P. is named for Sean O'Regan, M.D., an Irish pediatric kidney specialist who was the first to prove, back in the 1980s, that chronic constipation causes bedwetting. His published research also demonstrated that daily enemas safely resolve enuresis, encopresis, and chronic urinary tract infections. The guy was brilliant. (He still is, though he's now retired and living in Arizona.)

Once published, Dr. O'Regan's studies were largely ignored. When I dug up them up 25 years later, my mind was blown! I had already come to realize constipation causes virtually all bedwetting — that "deep sleep," stress, hormonal imbalance, an "underdeveloped bladder," and all the other popular theories are nonsense. But I hadn't known this fact was so well documented,

3 Dave Barry, "A journey into my colon — and yours." Miami Herald. Febr. 22, 2008. https://www.miamiherald.com/living/liv-columns-blogs/dave-barry/article1928847.html.

that these kids are so monumentally constipated, or that daily enemas are the only reliable remedy.

When it came to treating constipation, I wasn't as passive as many doctors are, but I also wasn't as tenacious as I should have been.

Dr. O'Regan's research changed my entire approach to treating enuresis and encopresis and dramatically increased my success with patients. Finally, I could help these kids! They could go on stress-free play dates and sleepovers. They could attend school without fear of having an accident in class.

Over the years, I have modified Dr. O'Regan's original regimen, hence the term "Modified" O'Regan Protocol, but his research remains the basis for my approach.

Now, I won't sugarcoat things: **M.O.P.** can be a tough road. It's not that enemas are traumatic — despite what doctors may tell you, enemas quickly become routine for constipated kids and bring them tremendous relief. As one mom put it, "My daughter asks for enemas and has increased confidence five-fold because she's not smelly. She used to ask me in a whisper if she smelled OK. Now THAT was traumatic, especially when you're in middle school."

Still, progress on **M.O.P.** can be slow, and setbacks are common. The regimen is time-consuming and requires a lot of trial and error, and certainly no 6th-grader wants to get an enema every night. Often, store-bought enemas won't do the job[4], and kids require homemade, large-volume enemas with stimulants such as glycerin (the **M.O.P.+** regimen), overnight olive-oil enemas (**DOUBLE M.O.P.**), or expensive pump systems.

Parents are astounded at how difficult it can be to dislodge hardened stool. As one mom in our support group posted, "I feel like I am chipping away at a cement block with a garden hose!"

Sometimes, even when the rectum is fully cleared out daily, it can take a year for a chronically stretched rectum to shrink back to size.

---

4 MA Levitt MA and A Peña. "Minimally invasive treatment of fecal incontinence and constipation in children." Minerva Chirurgica. April 2010; 65(2):223-34. https://www. ncbi.nlm.nih.gov/pubmed/20548277.

The stubborn nature of constipation in children makes a mockery of the idea that prune juice, more veggies, and Miralax can fix the problem.

What is PRE-M.O.P.?

Though the medical community continues to undertreat constipation in babies, parents are becoming more savvy. In recent years, I have received more clinic visits and email inquiries from parents of children under age 3 who are chronically constipated.

These parents grasp what may lie ahead for their children and are eager to resolve constipation before their kids start school. Many have found **M.O.P.** online and ask:

1) **Can I put my baby on the regimen? She's already showing serious signs of constipation.**

2) **Can I do M.O.P. without Miralax? I've heard reports of rage, anxiety, and OCD and don't want to give it to my child.**

My answers in short:

1) The full **M.O.P.** regimen is typically unnecessary for children who have not started toilet training or who have become constipated only recently upon learning to use the potty. A limited version, what I call **PRE-M.O.P.**, should suffice.

   PRE-M.O.P. has two key components: a daily osmotic laxative and a liquid glycerin suppository (essentially a small enema) given in the evening *on any day during which the child has either not pooped at all or appears not to have completely emptied*. Children under age 2 use a solid rather than liquid suppository.

2) Yes, you absolutely can treat chronic constipation in young children without Miralax.

   I don't oppose Miralax (an American brand name for PEG 3350) when parents are comfortable with it and children show no adverse symptoms. For most kids, PEG 3350 is effective and has negligible side-effects. However, I do take seriously reports of aggression, mood swings, compulsive behavior, and other neuropsychiatric symptoms parents have reported after giving their children PEG 3350. There is no reason to use this powder if you don't want to. You can choose from several effective alternatives.

Compared to the usual remedies, **PRE-M.O.**P. may sound excessive. Do you really need to give a baby laxatives and mini-enemas? I believe you do! That is, if you'd like to prevent your child from ever setting foot in an incontinence clinic like mine.

Just this week a mum in New Zealand emailed that she'd given her constipated 2-year-old laxatives since age 6 months, and it didn't solve the problem:

> *It works for a few months until she starts getting constipated again. Her bowel movements can be larger than an adult sized stool, which leaves her in tears. Now she holds on till she's at home, with both her stools and urine, which can be for hours at a time. Our paediatrician says it's fairly common and there nothing else we can do. I feel helpless for her. All bowel diseases have been ruled out.*

I hear this all the time! And her doctor is mistaken: There actually *is* something else she can do: **PRE-M.O.**P.

As I've mentioned, **PRE-M.O.**P. is primarily intended for children who have not initiated toilet training or who are new to toilet training and struggling to poop in the toilet. Potty training a constipated child is a frustrating and futile endeavor for all involved and will surely backfire. So, if you're in this boat, I recommend you stop training your child and implement Pre-**M.O.**P. before you resume.

If your child has already been toilet trained for a few months and continues to have accidents, I recommend the full **M.O.**P regimen, even if the child is under age 3. The key difference is that with **M.O.**P., you administer a liquid glycerin suppository or pediatric enema every single day for at least 30 days *no matter* *what* — not just on days when your child doesn't poop or doesn't fully evacuate. There are numerous other components of the program that pertain only to toilet-trained children.

It is essential to resolve your child's constipation completely and for several months before you begin or resume potty training, regardless of any deadlines your preschool has set. Part 6 provides guidance on toilet training children who've been through **PRE-M.O.P.**.

Coming Attractions

This book has two themes: 1) Be aggressive with treatment, and 2) Be patient as you work to fix constipation for good.

Do not set any timelines for resolving your child's withholding, for ditching diapers, or for putting all this poop business behind you!

Parents, understandably, are eager to halt laxatives once constipation appears to be resolved, but stopping too soon is a recipe for relapse. I recommend continuing laxatives and suppositories (when necessary) through potty training and well beyond — ideally through the beginning of kindergarten.

The book will provide guidance as you work to resolve your child's immediate constipation crisis, prevent a recurrence, move on to toilet training, and pre-empt the accidents that plague my patients.

Among the topics I'll cover:

- 18 signs of constipation, some subtle and not well known
- Why **PRE-M.O.P.** is more effective than the alternatives
- How to implement **PRE-M.O.P.** without Miralax
- When eliminating cow's milk is warranted
- Toilet training a child with a history of constipation

In addition, you'll get the perspective of parents who've been through **M.O.P.**, including some who are now implementing **PRE-M.O.P.** with their younger children in hopes of avoiding a repeat.

As one mom in this situation posted:

> *I learned my lesson with my older daughter, who's now 4 1/2. She was constipated at 1 year, but the doctor just told me to give her prune juice and more vegetables. She ended up with encopresis and enuresis and was having 10 accidents a day. It took 8 months on **M.O.**P. for her to get down to 1 accident. My baby showed signs of constipation at 6 months, and I started doing for her what I should have done with her sister: a laxative every day and suppositories on days she doesn't have a good poop. An incredible amount of poop comes out with the suppositories, and I can see she feels so much better. I will do anything not to have to deal with encopresis and enuresis with more than one child.*

You now have the benefit of these moms' hindsight. So, let's get started!

Glossary of Terms

The Vocabulary of Constipation

The world of constipation treatment has its own vocabulary! Here, in alphabetical order, are terms I use often in the book and in our **PRE-M.O.P.** and **M.O.P.** support groups. I explain these terms in greater detail elsewhere in the book.

Encopresis: Recurrent poop accidents, which often happen without the child noticing. Though encopresis (aka "enco") is often mistaken for a behavioral or psychological condition, it's actually caused by constipation. Children with encopresis cannot sense the urge to poop or fully evacuate because the rectum, stretched by stool build-up, has lost sensation and tone.

Enema: A treatment to stimulate a bowel movement by squeezing fluid into the rectum via a flexible plastic tube. Enemas typically prompt the child to poop quickly, often within a few minutes. Store-bought pediatric enemas (2.25 ounces) are half the size of adult enemas and can be purchased over the counter. They contain a mix of saline and phosphate and are more effective at cleaning out the rectum than oral laxatives.

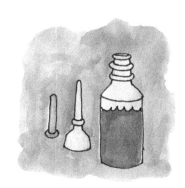

Enuresis: Involuntary wetting, either daytime or nighttime. Both daytime wetting and bedwetting are almost always caused by chronic constipation. The stool-stuffed rectum presses against and aggravates the bladder, triggering "hiccups" the child cannot control.

LGS: An acronym for liquid glycerin suppository, essentially a mini-enema. The bulb containing the liquid is the size of a grape, whereas a pediatric enema bottle is the size of an extra-large shot glass. For some kids, the phosphate in pediatric enemas causes a burning sensation whereas glycerin does not, though for some kids, phosphate produces more output than glycerin. In **PRE-M.O.P.**, you administer an LGS or enema on any day when the child does not poop spontaneously or does not appear to have fully emptied.

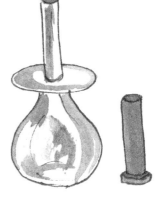

Osmotic laxative: An oral medication — in liquid, powder, or tablet form — that draws water into the colon to keep poop mushy, making pooping less painful. Effective laxatives include magnesium hydroxide (milk of magnesia), PEG 3350 (Miralax), magnesium citrate, and lactulose (sold by prescription in the United States but over the counter in many countries). Osmotic laxatives are taken daily throughout **PRE-M.O.P.** and ideally through the start of kindergarten.

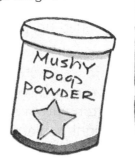
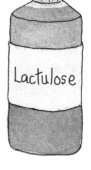

Rectum: The end of the colon. Normally, the arrival of stool in the rectum signals to the brain that it's time to poop, and the child empties. But if the child ignores this signal, stool begins to pile up. The rectum is not designed to store stool, and as the poop stockpile becomes larger, it can trigger extremely urgent or frequent peeing, enuresis, encopresis, and/or recurrent urinary tract infections. In children who have accidents, the diameter of the rectum is often greater than 6 cm, twice the normal diameter.

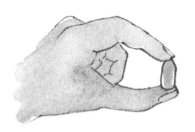

Solid glycerin suppository: A bullet-shaped dose of solid glycerin that is inserted in the rectum and, upon dissolving, stimulates a bowel movement. Solid suppositories take longer to work than liquid suppositories and tend to be less effective for older children. With **PRE-M.O.P.**, we recommend solid suppositories for children under age 2.

Spontaneous poop: A bowel movement that is not preceded by an enema or suppository — one that the child feels coming on and "just happens." A goal for children on **PRE-M.O.P.** and **M.O.P.** is to spontaneously poop every day.

Stimulant laxative: An oral medication that stimulates a bowel movement. Derived from the senna plant, stimulant laxatives such as chocolate-flavored Ex-Lax squares and Senekot liquid can be a helpful adjunct to **PRE-M.O.P.**, especially for toilet-training children who are extreme withholders. But these laxatives can cause cramping, and most kids on **PRE-M.O.P.** won't need them.

Helpful Resources

Books, Charts, and Support Groups

BedwettingAndAccidents.com: Our website, where you can access scientific studies, blog posts, and numerous free guides and charts for parents, children, educators, and medical professionals.

Private Facebook Support Group: An international Facebook group I run that mostly includes families implementing M.O.P. The group is not only private but also, in Facebook parlance, "secret," which means the group is not searchable to the public and is only visible to members. Members can post x-rays and unlimited questions. Members of this paid group includes parents, grandparents, and foster parents. For details, look under Support Services at BedwettingAndAccidents.com.

Private PRE-M.O.P. Support Group: A newer paid group, also private and secret, that is aimed at parents implementing PRE-M.O.P. Look under Support Services at BedwettingAndAccidents.com.

PRE-M.O.P. Tracking Chart. A chart to help you track your child's progress on PRE-M.O.P. A sample is included in this book. You can download the full-size chart under PRE-M.O.P. on our website.

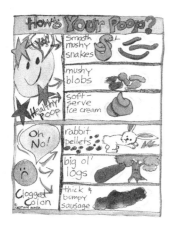

How's Your Poop? A free downloadable chart, available in English, that you can post in the bathroom to familiarize your child with the various sizes and shapes of poop. Look under Free Downloads on our website.

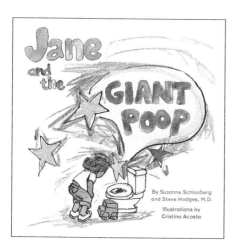

Potty Training Chart. A chart designed to help you spot signs of constipation as you toilet train your child. A sample is included in this book. You can download the full-size chart under Potty Training on our website.

A Letter to Preschool Directors and Teachers: A letter from me that you can copy from this book or download from our website (look under Potty Training) and hand to your child's educator. The letter emphasizes that children should not be required to be toilet trained by a certain age or date and explains why.

Jane and the Giant Poop: A rhyming book that can help toilet-training children learn what healthy poop looks like and why it's important to pee and poop often.

It's available in paperback on amazon or as a PDF on our website. Click on Books for Kids under Books & Guides.

Part 1

Diagnosing Constipation in Your Child

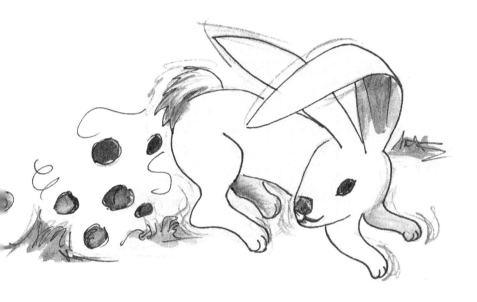

"For my son, constipation began between ages 1 and 2. I had no idea of the warning signs: the hiding to poop, big logs in his diaper, his face grimacing and showing effort to poop. I really wish I had known about the large logs."

You already know, of course, that your child is constipated — otherwise you wouldn't have bought this book. So kudos to you. You're on the ball!

However, in my experience, even parents who recognize constipation in their young children tend to underestimate, and therefore undertreat, the problem. When you're not attuned to all the clues, you may assume the issue is solved when, in reality, the flood gates are about to open. Sooner or later — usually sooner — your child relapses and you're back to square one.

Throughout the **PRE-M.O.P.** process you'll be tracking your child's progress, including the signs I describe in this section. It's critical to stick with the program until *all* indications of constipation have vanished and to keep your child's pooping output under surveillance for years (yes, *years*) so you can intervene at the first hint of backsliding.

"We started trying to potty train our son at around 3, and he flat-out refused to poop on the potty. I was told to give him prunes and lots of fiber, but it never really helped. He was on laxatives on and off but nothing consistent. I just thought that was the way he was, and that, as I'd been told, he'd grow out of it. Now he's 5 and has never pooped in the toilet. We've both been in tears many times over it."

Constipation in a baby can look very different from constipation in a 3-year-old. What's more, the signs can vary greatly from one child to the next. One toddler may writhe in pain before pooping and poop just twice a week; another may seem perfectly content and poop daily, though the size and consistency of her stools reveal that her pipes are epically clogged.

If you have a younger child or plan to have more children, knowing these signs will help you quell any problems before they worsen. Younger siblings of children on **M.O.P.** benefit greatly from their parents' new-found awareness.

For example, the mom of a bedwetting 7th-grader posted:

> *We started **M.O.P.** to help my 12-year-old son. Meanwhile, my 3-year-old was doing great with urinating in the toilet but was refusing to poop in it. I thought it was stubbornness and a behavior issue, so I continued to push him to sit and go in the toilet. In retrospect, that's when the constipation started. When I figured out he was constipated, I immediately started addressing the constipation. I truly feel it helped me avoid what I'm dealing with now with my 12-year-old.*

M.O.P. parents can spot constipation 10 miles away! They have to stop themselves from approaching random strangers and launching into, "I know this is none of my business, but I'm certain your child is suffering from chronic constipation. Do you know what a liquid glycerin suppository is?"

Of course, you might actually want to share your concern — as gently as possible! — to relatives or close friends. I'm on a mission to increase awareness of the signs of constipation, so perhaps you can help spread the word without alienating everyone in your orbit.

As I've mentioned, virtually all chronically constipated children have no underlying medical condition causing the back-up. For most kids, the red flags I describe in this chapter suggest nothing more than a clogged rectum that laxatives and suppositories can resolve. However, there are exceptions. Later in this section, I will cover a handful of rare medical conditions that cause constipation and that you should rule out in consultation with your doctor.

Constipation Redefined

Let's talk for a moment about what **_constipation_** actually means.

Many folks define the term as "infrequent pooping" or "pooping less than 3 times a week." But these definitions, as I'll explain, are unhelpful.

Then there's the definition offered by the North American Society for Pediatric Gastroenterology, Hepatology and Nutrition "a delay or difficulty in defecation, present for two or more weeks, sufficient to cause significant distress to the patient."[1]

This definition is fine as far as it goes . . . which, I believe, is not far enough. This characterization overplays the distress angle and allows for too much time to pass before trouble is suspected.

If a child, especially one who's eating solid food, delays pooping for more than a day — heck, poop is already piling up. If you wait two weeks before taking action, you've waited way too long, especially if this isn't your child's first go-around with a clogged rectum. With some kids, a single episode of painful pooping can be enough to set chronic constipation in motion.

Also, it doesn't matter whether the delay in defecation is "sufficient to cause significant distress to the patient." Distress should not be a deciding factor. All that really matters, in terms of diagnosis and treatment, is the delay.

While distress is often a sign of constipation, many children become so accustomed to painful pooping that they don't show, or even experience, "significant distress." I was constipated for my entire childhood, and though in retrospect, pooping was painful for me, I would never have considered myself in distress. I figured straining to poop was normal. Plenty of kids do.

To me, it's more helpful to define constipation as *not fully evacuating the rectum every day.*

I've stolen this definition from Dr. O'Regan's studies. In his papers, he noted that constipation is routinely overlooked because physicians associate the term with pooping frequency. In reality, he argued, the issue is the stretched rectum, caused by *incomplete evacuation.* **This is why, with PRE-M.O.P., you'll give your child a suppository not just on days when the child does not poop at all but also on days when the child appears to not to have fully evacuated.** Yes, that's a gray area; you can't

---

1 "Evaluation and Treatment of Constipation in Infants and Children: Recommendations of the North American Society for Pediatric Gastroenterology, Hepatology and Nutrition." *Journal of Pediatric Gastroenterology and Nutrition.* Vo. 43:3. September 2006. e10-e13. https://journals.lww.com/jpgn/fulltext/2006/09000/evaluation_and_treatment_of_constipation_in.28.aspx.

always distinguish a full poop from a partial poop, but you'll get a feel for it soon enough.

So how can you tell if your child is chronically constipated? Oh, there are so many ways!

For toilet-trained children with enuresis, I confirm constipation with an abdominal x-ray and measure the child's rectal diameter. (Stool in the rectum is what causes problems; stool elsewhere in the colon doesn't tell you much.) A normal rectum is no greater than 3 cm in diameter, same as those rubber bouncy balls that kids love and that drive parents nuts.

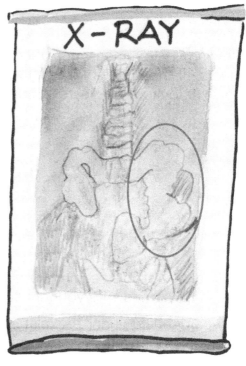

Abdominal x-rays are warranted in older children with enuresis. but for babies and toddlers you can detect constipation in other ways.

In a child with enuresis, the rectal diameter typically measures 6 cm to 9 cm. We're talking tennis ball (6.5 cm), baseball (7.5 cm), even softball (8.9 cm).

I x-ray my enuresis patients for several reasons. For example, it's helpful to have a baseline measurement for later comparison. If a child on **M.O.P.** continues to wet her pants, an x-ray typically explains why: the child's rectum is still clogged and stretched. Also, an x-ray can prove to skeptical parents and physicians that a child is actually constipated. Many doctors just don't believe it. They'll feel a child's belly, declare it "normal," and offer a debunked theory for why the child is wetting the bed.

Periodic x-rays are warranted for older children. but there is no reason to x-ray a baby or toddler. You can detect chronic constipation in numerous other ways if you know what you're looking for.

5 Red Flags in Babies

Following are common signs of constipation that begin in infancy. All these signs are common in older children, too, so be on the lookout for years to come.

Extra-large Poops

XXL poops are the number-one sign for kids of all ages, the reddest of red flags.

If your baby's stools seem impossibly large for a child so small, you can be darned sure your child is constipated.

Many parents are under the mistaken impression that mondo poops are a good sign. I've heard parents insist their child can't be constipated because she makes "big, healthy poops." But "big" does not equal "healthy." It just means stool has been accumulating in the rectum and has overstayed its welcome.

In toilet-trained children these giant poops can be toilet cloggers! One mom told me her daughter's titanic poops stopped up the toilet so often that she prohibited the girl from flushing unless an adult was standing by with a plunger.

"Looking back, my son's 'giant-human sized logs' were the warning signs about which we were clueless."

"At one point my son had a softball sized poop in his diaper. To this day I can't help but wonder: Did that really come out of him?"

"My daughter stood behind a curtain to poo. I remember having to coach her there doing a particularly big poo like she was giving birth!"

Once, this mom had to cut the poop down to size with a butcher knife!

It's stories like these that inspired our book *Jane and the Giant Poop*. Here's an excerpt from the book, which is fun and educational for kids age 3 and older.

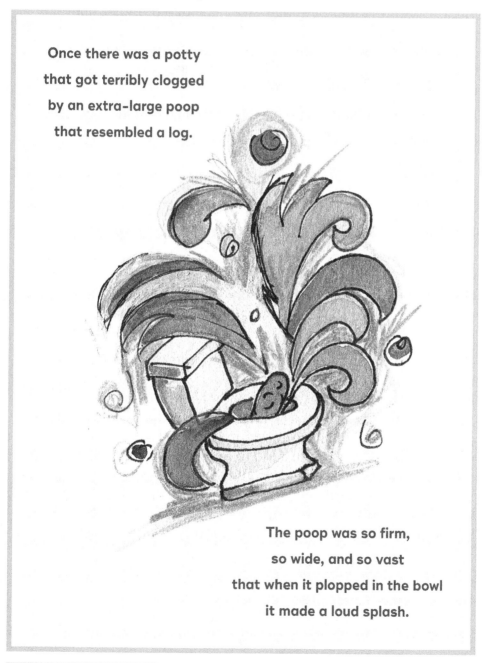

Once there was a potty

that got terribly clogged

by an extra-large poop

that resembled a log.

The poop was so firm,

so wide, and so vast

that when it plopped in the bowl

it made a loud splash.

Poops Formed Like Rabbit Pellets or Logs

Most folks don't realize stellar stool is a pile of mush, like pudding or a cow patty or a swirl of frozen yogurt. Soft, thin snakes are A-OK, too. But if your child's poop resembles a log, a turkey sausage, or — commonly in babies — rabbit pellets or marbles, your child is constipated!

Pellets are a telltale sign because as stool lingers in the rectum, water is sucked out of it and the hard, dry stool breaks into pieces.

In short, dry and firm: thumbs down. Moist and soft: thumbs up.

Straining or Crying to Poop

Grimacing in a newborn isn't necessarily cause for concern. The straining may be a sign of infant dyschezia, a condition that occurs in healthy infants and disappears within a few days.

Infants with this condition will strain and cry for at least 10 minutes, maybe even a solid half hour, while trying to poop. This is, of course, super stressful for parents. However, these babies' stools are normal, and the babies are not actually in pain. They just lack the coordination to crank out stool. Basically, pooping requires two things: ratcheting up intra-abdominal pressure and relaxing the pelvic floor. Some infants can't yet manage this duo, so they howl in an attempt to create force in their abdomen. Plus, when you're new to pooping, and to the world itself, the whole deal may just feel weird enough to trigger a crying frenzy.

Newborns with infant dyschezia don't require laxatives or any other treatment. Though my main message is "Be proactive!" in this particular case I urge parents to wait a few days before taking action. However, if a baby is more than a few weeks old and continues to strain, the baby is likely constipated

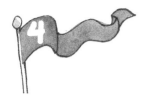

Bloody Stool or a Bloody Bottom

Passing a hard or large stool may cause anal tearing, sometimes to the point where the child bleeds a bit. So, stool may arrive with bright red blood on the edge, or you may notice blood on the diaper.

While this is alarming to parents, the tearing heals quickly, usually within a couple days, as long as you're able to soften the baby's stool. Do tell your pediatrician about the bleeding.

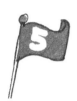

Infrequent Pooping

Pooping frequency, as I've mentioned, is a lousy indicator of constipation. Plenty of kids who poop every day are constipated. It's more important to consider what kids are pooping out — giant logs or dry pellets, for instance — than how often they are pooping.

However, if your child isn't pooping daily, that's a pretty bright red flag. Some doctors think it's fine if a child poops every other day. I am not one of those doctors! Though it's debatable whether an infant on breastmilk or formula needs to poop daily, I believe that any person who eats every day — including any child who has started

"My son became constipated when he started solids at 6 months. At 10 months he did not have a bm for 2 weeks. The doctor prescribed Miralax. I did not want to give it and eventually gave him probiotics. He always pooped daily, so I never knew he was so backed up until we did an x-ray when he was 7 and was still wetting at night. Now he's 8 and has daytime wetting, too."

on solid foods — should poop every day. A child who doesn't poop daily may be headed for trouble. A child who poops once or twice a week is already experiencing a major stool build-up.

Babies under age 1 poop, on average, 2.2 times a day, research suggests, so if a child that young goes even one day without pooping, a back-up has begun.[2] Children between ages 1 and 3 poop, on average 1.4 times a day, so for that age group, too, I'd be concerned about a child who does not poop every day, especially if the child is showing other signs of constipation.

7 Red Flags in 2- and 3-Year-Olds

The followings signs tend to surface around potty-training age but, like those listed in the previous section, apply to older children as well.

Hiding to Poop

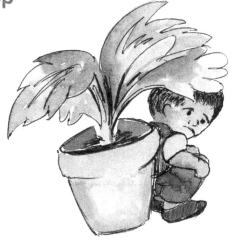

Some toddlers in diapers seek privacy to poop — they'll hide in a closet, behind the curtains, in a playhouse, behind the couch. Parents may be unsure what to make of this behavior. Some parenting coaches mistake it for a sign of readiness to potty train. In fact, in one article I read, a potty-training coach wrote that hiding signals that children "can tell that they need to poop before they actually go and have a better awareness about what's going on with their bodies."

2   Wendy S. Biggs and William Dery. "Evaluation and Treatment of Constipation in Infants and Children." *American Family Physician*, 1;73(3), Feb. 2006: 469-477. https://www.aafp.org/afp/2006/0201/p469.html.

Hiding may indicate some awareness, but it also indicates something more important: the kid is constipated! Which means the child is absolutely *not ready* to toilet train – quite the opposite.

Hiding to poop is common among constipated toddlers, but it's usually not the first sign of constipation, just one of many.

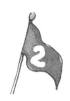 ## Skid Marks or Itchy Anus

Poop smears, aka "skid marks," in a diaper or underwear and the itching they cause are signs of constipation that tend to go unnoticed by parents. Once children are toilet trained, adults often interpret skid marks as a sign of poor wiping, but what these smears actually signal is the child hasn't fully emptied or has been trying to hold poop in. As one mom recalled, "I talked myself into thinking skid marks were just 'bad wiping' because I wanted so badly for that to be the reason. Now, I know better. I never stop checking for skids."

Poop smears are such a reliable sign of constipation that with **M.O.P.**, we consider them essentially the equivalent of a poop accident. In other words, if a child with encopresis has been accident free for a while, has tapered to twice-weekly enemas, and then has a skid mark, we recommend the child resume daily enemas — just the same as if he'd pooped in his pants.

 ## Belly Pain or a Distended Belly

I recently had a 4-year-old patient who, according to her mom, regularly complained of belly pain. But this mom didn't perceive the stomachaches as a problem; she simply considered them an indication it was time for her daughter to poop.

Whoa there! The "time to poop" signal is the urge we all feel in the rectum. By the time a child has a stomachache, that urge has been suppressed repeatedly, and excess stool has already stockpiled. It's a bit like using extreme thirst as a sign to drink a glass of water: By the time you feel parched, you're well past the point at which you should have hydrated.

Many doctors dismiss belly pain in children because the complaint is so common. But as with bedwetting, common does not mean normal! Not all children who are constipated experience belly pain or complain of discomfort, so you can't make any assumptions based on silence. In fact, one mom in our support group, whose bedwetting 11-year-old has been constipated since he was a baby, says her son has "never complained of abdominal pain or bowel movement pain, EVER!" — even though he has a history of stools the size of a Pringles can!

On the other hand, most children who frequently complain of stomachaches are constipated, as the stretching of the colon can cause discomfort. (Of course, the kind of achy tummy we're talking about is totally different from the sharp belly pain triggered by, for example, appendicitis.)

In some kids, the belly load full of poop is obvious. You can actually see the child's abdomen pooching out. One mom in our support group calls it "the poop belly." Now that she knows what she's looking for, she posted, "I see poop bellies everywhere. There is a stark difference between soft and pudgy and the firmer, distended poop belly."

However, in most constipated kids, the "poop belly" is not visible. Some of my most constipated patients have completely flat bellies and were pronounced "not constipated" by pediatricians who felt their abdomens. Their extreme constipation was confirmed by x-ray, not by my touch. Even the smallest, wiriest children can harbor truckloads of poop without anyone being the wiser. That's why it's so important to know the range of constipation signs.

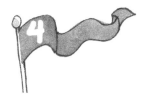

Decreased Appetite

Some kids feel so bloated and uncomfortable from hauling around their rectal cargo that they just don't feel like eating much. Often this lack of appetite goes unnoticed. It's only when the constipation is resolved and the child starts chowing down that the parents realize what had been going on.

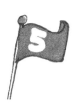

Diarrhea

Wait, what? How can loose, watery stool be a sign of constipation? Isn't constipation characterized by just the opposite: hard, dry poop? Well, yes. But often fresh poop oozes around the hard mound, and the end product resembles diarrhea. Parents get the impression the child is *anything but* constipated when the opposite is true.

While pellets and big logs are pretty reliable indicators of constipation, don't get complacent if you see super soft or runny poops. As one mom wrote, "I have found that the consistency of poop has nothing to do with how backed up my kiddo is. Her poops are all over the place. I know liquid stool can leak around a blockage, so I don't trust consistency as a guide."

Pooping More than Once a Day

In an article titled "I Can *Not* Get My Kid To Poop In The Damn Toilet," a frustrated mom seeks to solve the mystery of her 3-year-old's "refusal." She dismisses the idea that her son could be constipated: "Dealing with a steady stream of poop-filled diapers assures me that my son is having regular bowel movements."

But that "steady stream" is itself a sign of constipation!

More is not better. Yes, it's normal for infants to poop more than once a day. But in toddlers and older kids, pooping multiple times a day signals the child is not fully emptying, because when kids fully empty, they do not need to poop more than once a day. **The human body is designed for a single daily evacuation.**

As for the article author, she inadvertently confirms her son is constipated by describing the contents of his diapers: "the diarrhea poops, and the huge poops, and the tiny poop nuggets that always escape the confines of a soiled diaper."

Three smoking guns!

Reluctance to Poop in the Toilet

I refuse to use the term "potty refusal." This term implies the child is being obstinate, stubborn, willful — "refusing" to do what is asked, in protest of your parenting. In reality, these kids are fearful. Usually they fear pooping will be painful, as perhaps it has been for them in the past. However, some kids fear falling into the toilet or have a sensory reaction to the flushing sound, particularly the automatic-flush toilets in public restrooms.

When you initiate toilet training and your child is reluctant to poop in the toilet, this doesn't necessarily mean your child is constipated. Another possibility, quite common, is that your child simply isn't ready to toilet train. (I list the signs of readiness in Part 6.) However, if your child is around age 3, the typical age of readiness, and is averse to pooping in the potty, constipation is a good bet. Consider this sign in conjunction with the others listed in this section.

6 Red Flags in Toilet-Trained Children

A child who was constipated as a baby will always be at risk for a recurrence. I've had patients who suddenly started having daytime pee accidents in 4th grade, baffling their parents, who had long since forgotten their child was ever backed up.

But sometimes circumstances change — a kid transfers to a school with restrictive restroom policies, becomes less physically active, starts eating more junk food, or has a digestive illness — and constipation returns, triggering new and more severe symptoms. In most cases, the child was constipated all along but the symptoms were manageable. And since the parents had long since stopped chaperoning the child to the bathroom, they were none the wiser. Most parents of 4th graders have no idea whether their child is pushing out giant logs or how often their child poops. Certainly my own parents had no clue I was constipated.

Since your child will be prone to constipation in the future, it's important to know the red flags in older children. Also, though this book is targeted at parents of kids 3 and under, constipation often runs in families. Parents working to resolve constipation in young children may not even realize they have older kids who also are chronically constipated. While your baby's signs may be obvious to you, your older child's may not be.

In addition to enormous stools, belly pain, skid marks, and the other signs listed above, the following are telltale signs in toilet-trained children.

Urinary Frequency

I once read an advice column in which a schoolteacher wrote: "I have a student who will literally ask to use the bathroom 48 times in 4 hours. (I kept a tally.) This child does not have a medical condition. This child is not bored. This child just wants attention."

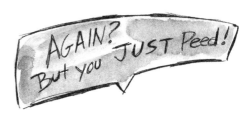

Hold up! This child likely does have a medical condition. It's called urinary frequency. The nerves that control the bladder essentially go berserk, sending premature — and terribly frequent — signals to the bladder that it's time to pee. In some cases, the mega-load of poop also crowds out the bladder, so it can no longer hold enough urine for substantial lengths of time.

Urinary frequency is particularly common in 4-year-olds, probably because it takes a year or two after potty training for the rectal clog to reach a critical mass — literally. But kids of all ages can develop this condition.

When they do, parents wonder, "How can a child possibly produce so much urine?" and may suspect the child has diabetes. It's true that frequent peeing is a sign of type 1 diabetes, but children with diabetes also experience other symptoms — hunger, weight loss, fatigue — that constipated kids don't. I've examined thousands of kids with urinary frequency, and exactly one tested positive for diabetes.

If a toilet-trained child has urinary frequency but not accidents, PRE-M.O.P. should suffice. But if a child has both frequency and enuresis, the full M.O.P. regimen is warranted.

Urinary Urgency

The same process that causes urinary frequency also triggers urinary urgency. the overwhelming need to pee RIGHT NOW. This second. Head directly to the toilet. Do not pass Go. Do not collect $200.

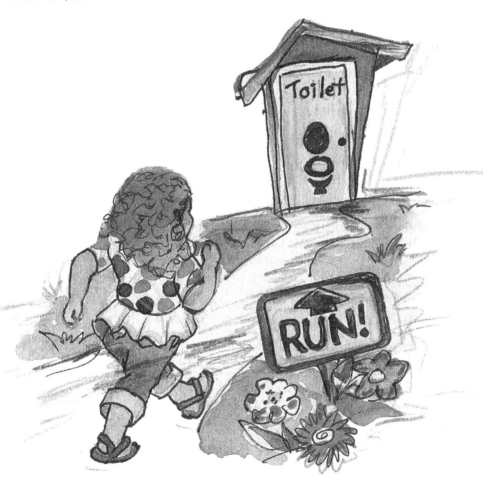

Bedwetting

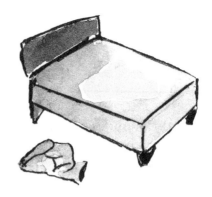

Bedwetting is not a mystery! As I've explained, virtually all cases are caused by constipation — not deep sleep, an underdeveloped bladder, an overproduction of urine, anxiety, or any of the other common explanations. While bedwetting often does run in families, that does not mean the wetting itself is hereditary; it's the tendency toward constipation that is inherited, along with the sensitivity of the bladder to interference from the stuffed rectum.

(For a detailed explanation of why "deep sleep" and the other theories don't hold water, read my blog post "To the American Academy of Pediatrics: Please Update Your Bedwetting Advice."[3])

It can take a long time for parents to recognize bedwetting as a problem, since it's usually not a condition that suddenly appears but rather is a condition that doesn't disappear. Also, many doctors tell families bedwetting is normal and not worthy of treatment until at least age 7. I've even worked with families who were told bedwetting is normal at age 11!

That's nuts. I strongly believe in treating bedwetting starting at age 4. You cannot assume a child will outgrow the condition. My teenage patients will tell you that! And research backs them up. As one study of 16,000 children showed, children who have both daytime and nighttime wetting are far less likely to outgrow bedwetting than children who wet only at night.[4]

3 Steve Hodges. "To the American Academy of Pediatrics: Please Update Your Bedwetting Advice." https://www.bedwettingandaccidents.com/singlepost/ 2018/05/09/To-the-American-Academy-of-Pediatrics-Please-Update-Your-Bedwetting-Advice.

4 CK Yeung, B. Sreedhar, et al., "Differences in characteristics of nocturnal enuresis between children and adolescents: a critical appraisal from a large epidemiological study." British Journal of Urology International, 97(5). May 2006: 1069-73. https:// www.ncbi.nlm.nih.gov/pubmed/16643494.

Keep in mind that bedwetting can surface even after many years of dryness. The medical community calls this "secondary bedwetting" and considers it a different condition from primary bedwetting (overnight wetting that has never gone away), often attributing it to stress or anxiety. In reality, it's the same condition and requires the same treatment. When you take a hard look at the histories of my "secondary" bedwetting patients, you inevitably see a long history of constipation that was overlooked.

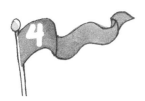

Daytime Pee Accidents

Though some doctors make a big distinction between daytime accidents and bedwetting, these conditions are in fact caused by the same process: a bladder gone haywire due to a clogged and stretched rectum.

Usually children with daytime wetting are more constipated than kids who wet only at night. However, I have numerous patients with daytime wetting who are dry at night. Their parents assume the accidents are behavioral — how could a kid go 10 hours overnight without peeing but be unable to hold it for an hour during the day? I know it seems impossible, but in some kids, that's just how constipation manifests. X-rays prove these kids are constipated.

Poop Accidents

Encopresis is always caused by an overflow of stool in the rectum, a fact that doesn't stop many doctors from telling parents it's a behavior issue. I've had countless encopresis patients referred to behavioral psychologists by their physicians or schools.

Encopresis tends to be more devastating to families than enuresis, but the good news is, it's easier to fix. Much easier.

While laxatives such as Miralax often make the problem worse — the softer poop just creates a big mess — daily enemas usually clear up encopresis within a month. However, it's critical that families complete the entire **M.O.P.** regimen (90 days at minimum), because any child constipated enough to have encopresis is very prone to a relapse. Many families get so excited when the poop accidents stop that they don't complete the protocol, and the accidents recur.

Chronic Urinary Tract Infections

I have patients as young as age 2 who regularly get urinary tract infections. Though their parents are often mystified, I'm never surprised, as chronic UTIs are caused by a common double whammy: holding poop and holding pee.

When a girl ignores the urge to poop, infection-causing bacteria in stool idle in close proximity to the outside world. They can colonize the perineum, the area between the vagina and anus, and eventually can make their way to the bladder. (In boys, the anatomy is different, so the same behavior does not result in UTIs.)

Here's how holding pee adds to the problem: When the same poop-holding girl squeezes her legs to override the urge to pee, the urge vanishes but the urine remains in the urethra, where the bacteria hang out. So, instead of getting flushed out, the urine picks up bacteria, allowing the bacteria to ride the urine back into the bladder. Next stop: UTI.

Antibiotics will clear up an infection but won't prevent a recurrence. Girls with recurrent UTIs need to clean out the rectum daily, ideally with enemas, and pee about every 2 hours.

Medical Conditions to Rule Out

I recently saw a 4-year-old patient who was having frequent pee accidents, a telltale sign of constipation.

Only this kid wasn't backed up. An x-ray showed his rectal diameter was completely normal and the rectum harbored no stool.

An ultrasound revealed the culprit: posterior urethral valves, extra membranes that develop in utero and block the flow of urine through the urethra, causing accidents and eventually, if not repaired surgically, bladder and kidney damage.

This disorder occurs in 1 out of 8,000 births, always in boys. It's almost always picked up on prenatal ultrasounds, but some cases slip by. I've seen the condition twice in my career.

Cases like these serve as a reminder that you can't make snap judgments. Virtually all my enuresis, encopresis, and UTI patients — more than 99% of them — are healthy kids who have no underlying medical cause for constipation. Still, there are exceptions, and while most congenital conditions are diagnosed at birth or shortly thereafter, occasionally the signs are missed.

Below I list congenital conditions that can cause constipation in very young children. This is not an exhaustive list. It highlights the more "common" of these uncommon anomalies.

In addition to the conditions listed here, diseases such as cystic fibrosis and hypothyroidism can cause constipation and incontinence. So can celiac disease, an autoimmune inflammatory disease of the small intestine spurred by eating gluten. In cases like celiac, where the root cause of constipation is a dietary intolerance, dietary changes don't usually fix the problem but are important for preventing a recurrence. When chronic constipation has already set in, treatment such as M.O.P. is usually needed to repair the rectum. When the cause is a neurological or anatomical condition, the fix is often surgical.

Hirschsprung's Disease

Children with Hirschsprung's disease are missing nerve cells from part of the colon and the rectum. So, instead of getting pumped along through the bowel, stool gets stuck.

When a newborn doesn't poop within 48 hours of delivery, that's a red flag for Hirschsprung's disease. Babies with Hirschsprung's typically have additional symptoms, such as a swollen belly, pencil-thin stools, failure to thrive, explosive and bloody diarrhea, and vomiting a green or brown substance. These children tend to land in the hospital frequently.

Though Hirschsprung's is usually diagnosed at birth, children with the "short-segment" version of the disease — meaning, they lack nerve cells only in the rectum — sometimes go undiagnosed until age 3 or even older.

Hirschsprung's disease occurs in about one in 5,000 newborns and is resolved by surgically removing part of the colon. I've never had a case in my clinic, though I encountered a child with Hirschsprung's disease when visiting the clinic of a colleague.

Congenital Anorectal Malformation

In about 1 in 5,000 children, the anus or rectum doesn't develop properly, and these kids have serious pooping problems that must be corrected surgically. Anorectal malformations are almost always diagnosed at birth and quickly corrected, although even with surgery these children may have difficulties pooping and need enema treatment.

Anorectal malformations include imperforate anus, where the opening to the anus is missing or blocked; anal stenosis, a narrowing of the anal canal; and an anteriorly displaced anus, where the anus isn't located in its normal position.

I've never seen a patient whose anorectal malformations were not already diagnosed and corrected surgically. When the rare case is referred to me, it's because the child has resulting bladder issues.

Spinal Cord Abnormalities

Children with nerve problems in their lower spine have abnormal bowel function, known as "neurogenic bowel," because of faulty communication between their brain and their bladder and bowels. As a result, their bowels move at a pokey pace. In addition, these children can't sense the rectum is full and/or can't fully empty the rectum.

Conditions that cause neurogenic bowel include spina bifida, which occurs when the spine and spinal cord don't form properly, and a related condition called tethered cord syndrome.

Spina bifida occurs in 5 or 6 out of 100,000 newborns and is almost always diagnosed before or just after birth. With these kids, part of the spinal cord is exposed through a gap in the backbone.

With tethered cord syndrome, the spinal cord, which normally floats freely inside the spinal canal, is stuck to the spinal canal and can become stretched and damaged. Telltale signs include a dimple or tuft of hair on the lower back and a lower spine that veers off to the side. These kids also tend to have poor reflexes or weakness in the legs.

I've seen plenty of patients with spina bifida for a variety of incontinence issues, but all were diagnosed long before visiting my clinic.

However, I've had two patients with tethered cord syndrome, a 4-year-old and a 13-year-old, who had not been diagnosed before their office visits. In both cases, their symptoms — encopresis, daytime enuresis, and bedwetting — suggested garden-variety cases of functional constipation.

It was only upon examination and further questioning that I discovered these kids were outliers. The 4-year-old had the telltale lower-back dimple and the off-kilter lower spine, and when I asked about leg weakness, his mom said, "Oh, yeah, his left foot sometimes goes numb."

The 13-year-old had no dimple and a spine that was barely deviated. I only thought to ask about foot weakness — which he did report — because his accidents came completely out of the blue during a growth spurt in puberty. Surgery to untether his spinal cord fixed the problem. The 4-year-old is headed for the same surgery.

You've probably heard the aphorism, common in medicine, "When you hear hoof beats, look for horses, not zebras." That is so true for enuresis and encopresis, but these two cases were important reminders that sometimes the hoof beats actually come from zebras.

How Your Child Became Constipated

When a child's anatomy is in order and everything else checks out medically, parents are often baffled as to why their children are chronically constipated.

Do you wonder how your child became so clogged at such a young age?

That's the topic for the next chapter.

Part 2

How Constipation Can Start So Early

"Knowing what I know now, I wouldn't have put a deadline on potty training, like our daycare did. I would have started slow with potty training."

It's no mystery why constipation is epidemic in the 21st century. The modern lifestyle serves to bog down our intestinal conveyor belt. As a species, we've engineered movement out of our lives, and we eat way too much highly processed food. And it doesn't help that instead of pooping in a squat, we sit on "comfort-height" toilets that position our bodies precisely opposite of what's optimal for easy evacuation. (More on that in Part 6.)

However, when your 8-month-old strains to poop, it's clearly not because he commutes an hour to work, spends all day hunched over his computer, binge-watches Netflix with his hand in a bag of Doritos, and poops on a 17-inch throne!

Clearly, something else is afoot.

In this part I'll explain how constipation develops in very young children. Typically, the condition emerges at one of three early stages and worsens with time and exposure to new circumstances, like entering preschool or grade school. Here's a look at what often happens at each of these stages.

Constipation in Newborns

When my youngest daughter was a couple weeks old, she'd strain like crazy to poop. She'd howl and shriek and wail . . . and then she'd unload totally normal, mustard-color mush. She was a classic case of infant dyschezia, the very temporary condition I describe in Part 1. Her straining stopped after a few days.

It's uncommon, but not unheard of, for newborns to have persistent trouble pooping. Every once in a blue moon the difficulty is due a congenital abnormality, such as tethered cord syndrome or Hirschsprung's disease. More often, it's because formula doesn't agree with the baby's digestive system.

For example, a mom in our **M.O.**P. support group posted that her daughter's constipation began shortly after her daughter's slightly premature birth and gradually worsened:

> *She was 3 weeks early and had jaundice. She was extra sleepy, so she wouldn't suck, and breastfeeding did not work. On formula, her poop was always formed, sometimes pellets or clay like consistency. By age 4 1/2, she was having lots of accidents. Miralax cleanouts and daily Miralax didn't help. Neither did senna tablets or timed potty breaks. Now, at age 9, she's on **M.O.**P.+. I wish I would have taken it more seriously from birth that she needed to be pooping every single day.*

Constipation at the Introduction of Cow's Milk or Solid Food

Though a small number of children experience constipation as newborns, a far more common scenario is for stool to start piling up between 4 months and 1 year, when babies wean from breast milk and/or formula and start drinking cow's milk, eating rice cereal, baby food, and other foods.

Breast milk, formula, and baby food promote mushy, seedy poop because they're loaded with water and are easily digested. But cow's milk tends to thicken poop. In some babies, this thickening comes as an unpleasant surprise; suddenly, pooping feels uncomfortable, and the baby starts withholding. This doesn't necessarily mean the baby has an intolerance or allergy to dairy. It may just mean the child is reacting to a new sensation in the body, brought on by the addition of new foods or beverages. Often, parents can successfully reintroduce cow's milk and yogurt months or years later, after treatment has enabled the child to overcome the holding habit. I've seen many cases like this.

> *"I noticed constipation from 4 months old, when he weaned from breast to formula, but it got really bad when he weaned at 6 months, which we now know was due to a cow's milk protein allergy. The key symptom was A LOT of crying and writhing about. We had to lift his legs and massage his tummy to get him to poo. He would scream as he passed it and often would bleed. Is it any wonder that at 5.5 years he still has chronic withholding behaviors?"*

But don't some kids have bonafide allergies to cow's milk protein? That's what several studies suggest, though other studies have found no connection. On the pages of prestigious gastroenterology journals, researchers have engaged in arguments that sound very polite and scientific but basically amount to: "Your study is crap" and "No, your study is crap."

Based on the published research and my own clinical experience, I believe that yes, some children do become constipated because of an intolerance to cow's milk. Is it an allergy? That's unsettled. But it's clear that for some children, cutting out dairy makes a huge difference. If your baby's constipation emerged around the same time you introduced cow's milk, I recommend eliminating dairy for about two weeks and closely monitoring your baby's stool size, consistency, and frequency during this time. Talk with your pediatrician about an appropriate replacement for cow's milk. If you see a significant improvement in your baby's pooping, you're well on your way to solving the problem. If a simple dietary change allows you to head off trouble, then consider yourself very lucky.

However, in my experience, it's usually not so easy. Even in studies that show great improvements when kids with documented cow's milk allergies stop drinking milk, plenty of kids remain constipated. This is probably because the withholding habit has already set in. Also, in many cases, a hard mass has already formed in the rectum, and eliminating cow's milk won't do anything to break it up and flush it out.

Even if eliminating cow's milk helps, you'll probably need to implement **PRE-M.O.P.** in addition to nixing dairy. The **PRE-M.O.P.** plan can get your child cleaned out and keep poop soft, so she (eventually) overcomes the fear of painful pooping. Eliminating dairy, meanwhile, may prevent constipation from recurring.

What if two weeks on a dairy-free diet does not clear up your child's constipation? I'd stop the elimination diet. If it's going to help, it's likely to help quickly. Some parents drive themselves and their kids berserk trying to avoid dairy even when it's clear the new diet isn't helping. Most children just aren't allergic to dairy, so while cow's milk intolerance is a real cause of constipation, it's not a common one.

More often, constipation in babies and toddlers develops at the introduction of solid food, particularly processed foods low in water content and fiber, the kind heavily marketed to parents of young children.

Fiber holds onto water as it passes through the bowel, helping stool remain soft. But Cap'n Crunch and goldfish crackers don't help the cause! In many kids, the shift from pureed peas to grilled cheese makes stools so thick that they become hard and painful to pass. In some babies, even organic rice cereal and pureed sweet potatoes can change stool consistency enough to trigger constipation. Plenty of babies who've never eaten a single goldfish cracker have become constipated, simply because of the way their body processes certain foods and reacts to a shift in stool consistency.

Think of it this way: For your whole life, squishy poop unassumingly makes its way out your bottom, and then suddenly a big lump of coal is attempting the same exit strategy. It's going to hurt, and you're going to remember it.

Even in babies, pooping is a voluntary activity. The urge to poop is triggered when stool travels from the intestinal tract into the rectum, where nerves alert the brain that it's evacuation time.

Normally, the child will heed that signal, contracting and then relaxing the external anal sphincter — what you probably think of as "the sphincter" but is actually one of two anal sphincters — and shoving poop out the door.

Ah, but what if the child doesn't want to poop? What if the child recalls a previous painful attempt and has no interest in reliving the experience? She'll instinctively tighten her sphincter and squeeze her gluteal muscles. This action shoves stool higher in the rectum, the opposite direction of where it's supposed to go, overriding the signal. **The urge to poop goes away, but the body's need to poop does not!**

So, stool keeps piling up. If the child repeatedly avoids pooping, the rectum stretches to accommodate the growing cargo load and ultimately loses propulsive power and sensation.

Meantime, the stockpile becomes bigger, drier, firmer, and more painful to pass. It's a vicious cycle: the child avoids pooping out of a fear of pain, which leads to even more avoidance and a greater backlog. The kid never wants to poop. But eventually, the load becomes so big that at least some of it simply must exit. That's when you observe the grimacing, sobbing, and squirming.

I've known parents so desperate to ease their sobbing babies' pain that they've resorted to digging into the child's bottom with the end of a spoon and scooping out the offending mass of rock-hard poop. I don't recommend inserting hard instruments into a child's bottom, but a gentle finger is okay if necessary. I've done it on plenty of patients.

This scenario plays out over and over in babies and toddlers. So, by the time these little ones begin toilet training, the vicious cycle is well established, and these kids are already at a huge disadvantage.

Potty training is not going to go well, no matter how many stickers or M&Ms you offer and no matter how many times your preschool reminds you that your child must be toilet trained by September.

Constipation When Potty Training Begins

Potty training is prime time for constipation to develop in kids — even kids who love veggies, guzzle water, and have been super poopers their whole lives. This is usually because, pain or no pain, kids ages 2 and 3 don't put pooping high on their daily agendas. They're far more interested in Play-Doh, finger painting, and miniature race cars. Also, as I've mentioned, some kids fear falling into the toilet or have a sensory reaction to the flushing sound.

Once kids are introduced to the toilet, they make some enlightening discoveries: They can control when they poop, and they can override the urge with some timely squeezing! Many of them capitalize on these newfound powers and delay pooping on a regular basis. Pretty quickly, a child who was dropping cow patties every day like clockwork is straining to shove out a big, hard log a few days a week. Constipation has commenced!

But parents, celebrating the prospect of a diaper-free future, haven't a clue.

Things go further awry when children feel pressure to master toilet training quickly.

Sometimes the messages are subtle. For example: "Yay! You're such a big boy! You didn't have any accidents!" Other times, the mandate is more overtly presented: "Hey, buddy — you're old enough to be out of diapers by now" or

"I think I was in some sort of weird denial regarding the chronic- ness of my son's constipation. I was an idiot and even weaned him off of Miralax. Daycare literally refused to inform us whether he pooped or peed. We thought he was pooping there, and they thought he was pooping at home. I couldn't get straight answers from anyone, especially my 3-year-old, and BOOM, one day I find he has rabbit pellets and blood in his diaper."

"Knowing what I know now, I would have switched daycares and not let them dictate my parenting. I wouldn't have put a deadline on potty training, like our daycare did. I would have started slow with potty training."

"If you're not potty trained by September, they won't let you into preschool."

The message children internalize is not, "The most important thing is for me to poop when my body tells me it's time" but rather, "If I stay dry, I will make all these grown-ups happy."

Sometimes parents are in a hurry because they've heard there's a "window of opportunity" to train, between age 20 and 30 months. As the author of one book asserts, "If you miss the window, you'll end up with a potty refuser."

This is a false and harmful misconception!

In other cases, potty training is hurried because the child's preschool has set a "toilet trained by 3" deadline. Preschool deadlines are particularly insidious. The message they send to kids is, quite literally, *Do not have an accident. Or else.*

One mom showed me the policy at her child's school: "If a child has multiple accidents in a day or over a period of days, and we realize a child is not fully toilet trained, we may ask that parents keep the child home for a week or two to complete his/her toilet learning." If the child continues to have accidents, the policy states, the family may be asked to leave school. The policy is "firm," according to the school, and is based on "best practices."

I can assure you it is not a "best" practice to suspend a child from school for failure to stay dry! It is a dreadful practice. Sending kids home for a week to work on their potty skills is like sending dyslexic children home for a week to work on their reading. It's going to fail, because these kids' issues have nothing to do with lack of training.

Another preschool's toileting policy puts a premium on the child's "willingness and cooperation" to use the toilet. The implication is that a child who sits on the toilet but won't pee or who pees on the floor is uncooperative. This notion is misguided, to say the least.

One of my patients was escorted off the premises of her preschool, along with her mom, after she had wet her pants more than the mandated limit of 8 times per month. The principal had told the child's mom that the 3-year-old had "had enough chances." The mom told me: "They acted like she was some kind of criminal."

When a child has a history of constipation, as this child did, the added pressure is going to backfire big time.

Even when kids arrive at preschool with a Ph.D. in toilet training and even when their teachers are kind and patient, as most preschool teachers are, simply being in a new environment can trigger or exacerbate constipation.

For many kids, preschool is the first time they're spending the day, or half a day, without family around. They may not feel comfortable interrupting their teacher during story circle to announce they need to go potty or may not want to climb out of the fort they've just built and venture over to the toilet.

They may decide it's just easier to squeeze that stool back where it came from and save pooping for another day!

Even 2- and 3-year-olds who don't attend preschool often become constipated during the potty-training process because they're reluctant to poop in unfamiliar places, like at the park or the supermarket. If that's where they are when the urge strikes, they may just ignore it. When a child will poop only at home, that's a prescription for trouble.

What's more, most constipated children don't tell their parents or teachers they're having difficulties. Usually they themselves don't know something is amiss, especially if painful poops are all they've experienced. So, the rectal pile-up goes undetected.

The younger and more immature kids are when they start potty training, the less likely they are to heed the urge to use the toilet. This is true even for children who train easily, like when Mom says, "She practically potty trained herself!"

In fact, my research, discussed in Part 6, shows that children who begin toilet training before age 2 have triple the risk of developing chronic constipation and enuresis compared to children who train between ages 2 and 3. This does not mean kids who start training at age 2 1/2 are out of the woods. There's no bright line that separates an inappropriate age from an appropriate age to train. What matters most is the child's maturity, not age.

Another reason not to rush toilet training: the earlier a child potty trains, the more months or years she has to develop the holding habit and develop chronic problems. This is a fact preschools don't consider when setting their deadlines.

A Full-Blown Constipation Crisis

So, there you have it — the litany of reasons children can become so constipated at such a young age.

Some children experience a triple whammy: They're prone to constipation as infants, they become more clogged at the introduction of solid food, and they're overwhelmed by the subtle or not-so-subtle pressures to toilet train in time for preschool. For these kids, potty-training brings on a full-blown constipation crisis. Yet when they visit the doctor, they're prescribed prune juice and veggies.

Ultimately, it doesn't matter whether your child became constipated at 6 months or 26 months. The buildup of poop can lead to all sorts of bladder and bowel problems, and it's important to resolve them now — before your child heads off to kindergarten and faces even steeper challenges.

Part 3

Prune Juice and Fiber Won't Cut It: The Case for PRE-M.O.P.

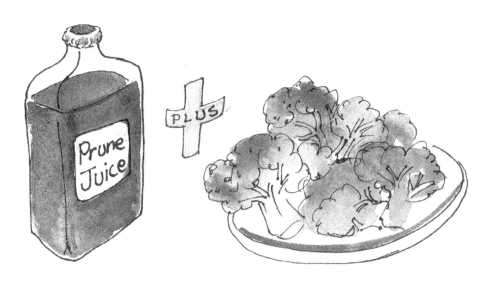

"At 6 months, the general practitioner refused to give him a laxative and told me to up his fiber and give him prune juice and lots of water. This was a weaning baby whose main foodstuffs were pureed fruit and vegetables!"

Let's say your 2-year-old has red, swollen gums and brown spots on her teeth, and, concerned by these symptoms, you take her to the dentist. No dentist on the planet is going to say, "Well, she's in the early stages of tooth decay, but eh, don't sweat it. Try cutting down a bit on the sugar."

Not gonna happen!

Instead, the dentist is going to sound the alarm about oral hygiene and sugary drinks, explaining that left unchecked, tooth decay in baby teeth can lead to decay in adult teeth, infection, speech difficulties, and other major problems that can follow your child into adolescence and adulthood.

But if your 2-year-old shows up at the doctor with just-as-obvious signs of constipation? The doctor is likely to say, "Don't worry — she'll outgrow it" and recommend she eat more fiber.

That's what has happened to numerous moms in our **M.O.P.** support group. Never mind that the consequences of undertreating constipation are potentially just as painful, damaging, and expensive as undertreating tooth decay — and a lot more embarrassing and stressful for the child.

For example, one mom, who recognized serious constipation signs in her 6-month-old son, posted:

> *The general practitioner refused to give him a laxative and told me to up his fiber and give him prune juice and lots of water. This was a weaning baby whose main foodstuffs were pureed fruit and vegetables! When he was 1½, I took him to the doctor again and was told he was 'too young for laxatives.' I took him again at around 3 years, when soiling started, and was finally given a laxative. I insisted on a referral to paediatrics just before he turned 4 and have repeatedly been told to use Miralax and pico sulfate [a stimulant laxative]. We've given up on our healthcare system and are going it alone.*

At every stage, this mom was prescribed the least helpful treatment possible, on some vague theory that more aggressive treatment was unwarranted at best or, at worst, unsafe.

Given the reluctance of physicians to treat constipation seriously, don't be surprised if you hear from your doctor that **PRE-M.O.P.** is "too aggressive," "too invasive," or "unnecessary." Though most babies have stellar diets, the medical community seems convinced that an even more spectacular diet is the solution.

I cannot tell you how many of my patients' parents have been scolded by their physicians for following **M.O.P.** or even **PRE-M.O.P.** If you experience push-back, consider this advice from a mom who did **M.O.P.** with one child and is currently doing **PRE-M.O.P.** with another:

"It is so hard to ignore a doctor that has studied so much about the human body, but they do get it wrong sometimes. Medicine is a practice, and the human body is too complicated. I just follow my instincts as a mom. First, I hear the advice. If it makes sense, I go for it. If it stops making sense I stop."

I'm in favor of taking a conservative approach in medicine. Though I'm a surgeon, I never take surgery lightly and always look for ways to avoid it. But laxatives, suppositories, and enemas are not surgery. They are not risky. Nor are they abusive or traumatic.

In the next section I will explain why aggressive treatment for constipation is both necessary and safe, even for babies, and how the **PRE-M.O.P.** approach stacks up against alternatives commonly prescribed by doctors.

The Origins of **M.O.P.**

A big reason doctors undertreat constipation in babies is that unlike dentists, who universally connect early tooth decay with future health problems, doctors tend to overlook the connection between early constipation and future bowel and bladder problems.

Many physicians don't recognize that constipation is both chronic and progressive and is the direct cause of enuresis and encopresis.

Sean O'Regan was not the first person to recognize this connection, but he was the first to prove it scientifically and to show that enemas resolve the problem. His story is remarkable.

Back in the 1980s, when Dr. O'Regan was a young doctor raising three boys in Montreal, his 5-year-old was wetting the bed every night. Often the boy would wake his parents. Dr. O'Regan, accustomed to operating on minimal sleep, would get the elbow from his wife to help their son change his pajamas and sheets. The boy was self-conscious about the wetting and didn't want to sleep anywhere but home. His bedwetting was causing tension in the family.

Dr. O'Regan was bewildered by the boy's bedwetting, since his other two sons had achieved overnight dryness around age 3. At the time, bedwetting children were assumed to have either psychological problems or anatomic anomalies, such as an excessively narrow bladder neck. Dr. O'Regan did not accept either explanation and went searching for answers at the renown McGill University Medical Library.

He was intrigued by what he found: studies dating back to the 19th century documenting that severely constipated children had a high rate of urinary problems. Research from the 1960s showed that kids with Hirschsprung's disease — the congenital disorder I describe in Part 1, in which colon nerve cells are missing — typically developed urinary problems. It was clear: peeing and pooping are closely related.

This was not common knowledge. Historically, the urinary and digestive systems were considered separate. I mean totally unrelated, like a home's plumbing and electrical systems.

Dr. O'Regan felt he'd struck gold.

Next, he asked a colleague to test his son for constipation using a procedure called anorectal manometry. This test, considered the gold standard, is not super fun. A small balloon is inserted into the child's bottom and gradually inflated; the more inflation the child can tolerate, the more the rectum has been stretched by stool buildup. A child with normal rectal tone will detect the balloon when it's inflated with just 5 ml to 10 ml of air, whereas a severely constipated child might not notice any sensation until the balloon is inflated with 40 ml of air. The O'Regan boy's results were astounding: Even when the balloon was fully inflated, to 110 ml, the size of a tangerine, Dr. O'Regan's son felt no discomfort.

Dr. O'Regan's colleague told him: "The boy's got no rectal tone."

At that point, Dr. O'Regan turned to the only reliable treatment for severe constipation: enemas. (Miralax wasn't even approved by the FDA until 1999, and back in the 1980s, doctors didn't typically consider enemas "abusive" or "traumatic," as many do today.) Dr. O'Regan gave his son one enema every night for a month, then every other night for a second month, and then twice a week for a third month. The boy would read *Winnie the Pooh* on his bed while awaiting the urge to poop.

Within two months, the boy had stopped wetting the bed. Shortly after that, Dr. O'Regan and colleagues launched a series of studies on local children with enuresis, encopresis, and chronic urinary tract infections. They found these kids weren't just slightly constipated; their rectums, like the O'Regan boy's, were severely stretched. The three-month enema regimen Dr. O'Regan had given to his son worked extremely well for these patients.

For example, in a 1985 study, Dr. O'Regan tracked 47 girls, average age 8, who had both recurrent UTIs and severe constipation. Most of these girls also had enuresis and/or encopresis. Within three months of starting the enema regimen, 44 of the 47 girls had stopped having UTIs. Among the 21 patients with encopresis, 20 had stopped having poop accidents. What's more, 22 of the 32 bedwetting girls were dry overnight and an additional 7 had seen dramatic reductions in wetting. Among the three girls who didn't improve, two said they had not followed the enema regimen as instructed.

Dr. O'Regan published several other studies that confirmed the direct connection between constipation and accidents. (They are posted in full on our website, bedwettingandaccidents.com.)

Yet today you will read online and possibly hear from your doctor that the cause of bedwetting is a mystery. On its website for parents, healthychildren.org site, the American Academy of Pediatrics lists eight "possible causes" of bedwetting, including deep sleep, an underdeveloped bladder, and hormonal imbalance. Six of these causes are unsupported or disproven by science.

Constipation is on the list, so that's a plus. Yet, in the treatment section, the AAP does not recommend treating constipation as a bedwetting treatment! That's like saying running too much causes stress fractures but failing to recommend running less as a remedy. (The only other proven "cause" on the AAP's list is an underlying medical condition, such as those I describe in Part 1.) I debunk all of these bogus causes, one by one, in my blog post "To the American Academy of Pediatrics: Please Update Your Bedwetting Advice."[1]

At any rate, I bet your doctor has never heard of Dr. O'Regan. I had not heard of him myself, until experiences with my own patients prompted me to delve more deeply into the scientific literature. That's when I came upon his studies and called him to learn more about the origins of his research.

I did learn in medical school that constipation is the main cause of bedwetting and accidents, but I did not grasp how monumentally constipated kids with enuresis are or how difficult it is to resolve chronic constipation once the vicious cycle has taken hold.

For several years I advocated Miralax as a satisfactory treatment for enuresis — a high-dose cleanout followed by many months of maintenance — even though I knew from experience that oral laxatives were less effective than enemas. Since it's easier to hand a child a glass of water mixed with a powder than to insert a tube into a child's bottom and most parents are averse to giving enemas, I figured it was reasonable to try the easier method first.

I no longer think that's reasonable.

Given the serious consequences of unresolved constipation, I now think it's imperative to do what works rather than to settle for what's easy.

My own research and experience show laxatives alone are not up to the task of cleaning out a rectum that's been chronically clogged and stretched and is so stretched as to be causing accidents. In fact, based on my clinical experience, I've ramped up Dr. O'Regan's protocol.

1   https://www.bedwettingandaccidents.com/single-post/2018/05/09/To-the-American-Academy-of-Pediatrics-Please-Update-Your-Bedwetting-Advice

Our kids' diets are more highly processed today than they were in the 1980s, physical activity levels are lower, and there's more pressure to potty train to meet preschool deadlines. Also, many school bathrooms are scarier and dirtier than they were in the 1980s.

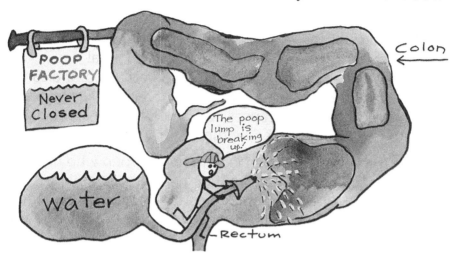

Dr. O'Regan showed daily enemas are safe and highly effective.

In response to these trends, I modified Dr. O'Regan's regimen to keep the rectum clear longer and to make pooping easier. I recommend daily enemas for *at least* 30 days, tapering only after the child has completed 30 enemas AND has remained dry for at least 7 consecutive days. I find many children need to extend daily enemas well beyond 30 days before they start tapering. Also, I recommend a daily osmotic laxative in addition to enemas.

I have found this regimen to be very successful. This is the protocol my clinic used in a study published in *Global Pediatric Health*[2]. We tracked 60 patients, ages 4 to 11, who typically wet their pants daily. Forty of these patients followed standard therapies, including daily Miralax, a pee schedule, and, in some cases, medication. Another 20 patients agreed to daily enemas for at least 30 days before tapering, plus daily Miralax. The results: After three months, 30% of the patients treated with standard therapies reported they'd stopped wetting, compared with 85% of the enema patients.

2 S.J. Hodges, M. Colaco, "Daily Enema Regimen Is Superior to Traditional Therapies for Nonneurogenic Pediatric Overactive Bladder," *Global Pediatric Health*, March 4, 2016: 3: 1–4. https://www.ncbi.nlm.nih.gov/pmc/articles/PMC4905156/.

A close look at the data explains why enemas worked better. The average rectal diameter in both groups was greater than 6 cm at the start of the study. Three months later, the rectums of the 40 patients treated with standard therapy remained stretched, to 5 cm on average, still 2 cm wider than normal.

But the rectums of the enema group had rebounded dramatically — to 2.15 cm, on average. That's a completely normal measurement. Enemas very obviously do a better job of cleaning out the rectum and of keeping it clear so it can heal. Miralax, as I've mentioned, often just causes soft stool to ooze around the large, hard mass clogging the rectum.

What about the three children in our enema group who did not stop wetting their pants? Unlike their peers, these patients were still stuffed with poop, according to our follow-up x-rays. Pediatric enemas simply weren't powerful enough to clear them out. For kids like these, I recommend more robust treatments such as large-volume enemas.

Parents are often stunned that after 30 consecutive days of enemas their child is still wetting every night. Many parents insist that I got it wrong — that constipation can't possibly be triggering the accidents. But then we'll take an x-ray, and the results will show the reality: the child's rectum is still chock full of poop.

Meanwhile, doctors are telling families to use more and more and more and more Miralax! And more!

How **M.O.**P. Led to **PRE-M.O.**P.

How does all this relate to babies and **PRE-M.O.**P.?

My experience with young children tells me that an aggressive approach is just as important for babies and toddlers as it is for older kids.

However, because babies and toddlers haven't been constipated as long, their rectums aren't as stretched. So, it's not as difficult to reverse course. It's usually enough for younger children to have a suppository or pediatric enema inserted only on days when they either don't poop spontaneously or appear to have not fully evacuated (in other words, if they barely poop).

For particularly clogged younger children, this may well mean they need a suppository or enema every day for a few weeks. Others may need the suppository a few times a week.

The suppository triggers the exodus of larger, harder masses of stool that may not budge with laxatives alone. Meanwhile, the daily laxative keeps stool soft by drawing water into the intestines. When stool is soft day after day, your child will eventually get the message that pooping is not painful and stop withholding.

I think that if more doctors understood how chronic constipation causes enuresis and how difficult it is to heal a chronically enlarged rectum, they'd be more supportive of a robust approach, not just for children with enuresis and encopresis but also for kids headed in that direction.

Instead, they tell parents that the insertion of a suppository or enema is "traumatic" and even belittle parents who choose this route.

One mom in our support group was told by a pediatric GI doc that enemas are dangerous to do frequently. She posted:

> " Doctors are so scared of enemas that they prefer your toddler go at least 3 days without pooping before getting a liquid glycerin suppository, and at least a week before getting an enema. My children were on adult doses of Miralax for long periods of time, and the situation kept getting worse. My son would only ever poop diarrhea, and he could hold in diarrhea for about a week, every week. Now that I see what a large volume of perfect consistency poop comes out of a child when they are having a bowel movement daily, I'm shocked most doctors are so comfortable with letting kids go an entire week without pooping, over and over and over again. "

I firmly believe rectal therapy is necessary. If a child is not fully evacuating every day, stool is piling up. Period. You don't want to wait until the mass becomes enormous! Suppositories and enemas will flush out dry, impacted stool. Prune juice and veggies won't. In the next section I consider the popular remedies that fall short.

PRE-M.O.P. v. the Alternatives

The most common remedies for constipation are dietary. To some extent, this makes sense. After all, what goes in affects what comes out. But this does not mean dietary changes and nutritious eating will clear out pipes that are chronically clogged. In most cases, dietary remedies are more helpful for preventing a recurrence of constipation than for cleaning out a clogged rectum.

Here's a look at the most popular remedies for babies and young children.

- **Prune juice and pear juice:** Prune and pear juice are the go-to constipation remedies for babies. These juices do have somewhat of a laxative effect because they contain sorbitol, a natural sugar alcohol that helps draw water into the intestines, softening stool. But juices aren't laxatives!

  They're just not potent enough to resolve the problem in most chronically constipated children, no matter how much the child drinks. Besides, juice is loaded with sugar, and for nutritional and dental reasons, guzzling juice isn't a good habit for any baby or toddler to start. I don't think there's any harm in giving a young child a few ounces a day of sorbitol-rich juice, but it's unlikely to clear up chronic constipation.

- **More fruits and vegetables:** I am never, ever opposed to anyone eating more fruits and vegetables. Fruits and veggies are the best! Children should eat plenty of produce every day, whether it's fresh, frozen, or canned. These foods are packed with fiber, which adds bulk to poop and helps speed up its transit through the colon, and they contain lots of water, which helps lubricate stool and ease its journey through the tunnel.

  Some 95% of children (and adults) don't get the

recommended daily amount of fiber[3] — 19 grams for children ages 1 to 3 and 25 grams for children ages 4 to 8. So, loading up on apples, berries, green beans, and broccoli will help kids meet that recommendation and will serve them well as they go through potty training, school, and life. But fruits and veggies, like juices, cannot dislodge a hard mound of stool impacted in a baby's rectum.

- **Fiber supplements:** Strawberry-flavored fiber gummies are not a great way to compensate for not eating strawberries. For a child averse to eating fruits, vegetables, and whole grains, fiber supplements can be helpful, but they are not a solution to chronic constipation and won't help your child develop healthy eating habits. There's no shortage of terrific websites devoted to helping families eat more nutritiously, so I'd start there rather than aim to get your child's fiber from a bottle of gummies.

- **Drink more water:** Fluid helps lubricate stool so it can move at a jaunty pace through the intestines. So, if your child has been weaned from breastmilk or formula and is not drinking plenty of water each day, by all means, get that child a fun sippy cup or water bottle and encourage frequent sipping. But water, like juice and veggies, will not empty a clogged rectum. If these remedies worked, I would not be writing this book.

- **Probiotics:** Probiotics are live microorganisms intended to enhance the trillions of "good" bacteria in your digestive system, the "gut microflora" that help protect against intestinal infections and possibly disease. This does not mean probiotics function as laxatives. I know many people swear by probiotics as a constipation remedy, but research does not support a laxative benefit. Probiotics may help restore the gut after a viral or bacterial illness that causes diarrhea, but again, if probiotics were a magic bullet for constipation, we'd know it!

3 Diane Quagliani and Patricia Felt-Gunderson, "Closing America's Fiber Intake Gap," *American Journal of Lifestyle Medicine,* 2017 Jan-Feb; 11(1): 80–85, https://www.ncbi.nlm.nih.gov/pmc/articles/PMC6124841/.

- **Eliminating dairy:** For constipated children with an intolerance or allergy to dairy, eliminating cow's-milk products is likely to help, often in a big way. But not always. Some dairy-intolerant children quickly learn to associate pooping with pain, so even after you eliminate the offending foods from their diet, they are still prone to withholding and need an aggressive regimen such as **PRE-M.O.P.** or **M.O.P.** There's no downside to eliminating dairy from your child's diet for a couple of weeks and noting any changes. But if cutting out dairy is going to help, it'll help quickly. I don't recommend prolonged elimination diets for kids who don't exhibit dairy intolerance, which is . . . most kids.

- **Eliminating gluten:** Removing gluten from the diet almost never helps. Unless your child has been diagnosed with celiac disease or another condition that directly connects gluten intake with digestive problems, I would not recommend this remedy.

Yes, Laxatives Are Safe for Babies

Many parents worry it's "not natural" to give laxatives to babies and toddlers, and many doctors steer clear of recommending laxatives for children that young (though for older kids, many of these same doctors don't hesitate to prescribe massive amounts of Miralax).

My take: It's not "natural" for a child to carry around a cargo load of poop, and the sooner the child gets cleaned out, the sooner she can get back to her "natural" state. Laxatives are safe, even for babies, and work a lot better than prune juice, high-fiber foods, and the other popular remedies covered in the previous section.

Osmotic laxatives far outperform juices and veggies in drawing water into the colon to make poop mushier and help it slide through. These laxatives are not habit forming and can be used for extended periods of time — even years, if necessary.

The osmotic laxatives most commonly used with **M.O.P.** and **PRE-M.O.P.** are PEG 3350 (Miralax), lactulose, magnesium hydroxide (milk of magnesia), and magnesium citrate. I discuss the differences among them in Part 4. The side effects for all these laxatives, mainly gas and nausea, tend to be mild or non-existent.

Miralax, however, is controversial. This powder is commonly prescribed by physicians worldwide, and studies on PEG 3350 in children have not detected any safety risks. At the same time, many parents have reported their children developed rage, anxiety, and other worrisome neuropsychiatric symptoms after taking PEG 3350, as I discuss in Part 4.

Some children respond better to certain laxatives than others, and I do not advocate giving children anything that makes them uncomfortable (or worse). I suggest experimenting with some or all of the laxatives listed in Part 4 to see which are most effective for and appealing to your child.

Osmotic laxatives are different from stimulant laxatives, like chocolate Ex-Lax squares or Senekot liquid. Stimulant laxatives are derived from the senna plant and stimulate the intestinal muscles to contract and squeeze out the idle poop. Stimulant laxatives come in liquid or chewable forms and are frequently used with **M.O.P.** For some kids, they're a game-changer. Like osmotic laxatives, stimulant laxatives are not habit forming and are safe for children, but they can cause cramping, especially in higher doses.

Compared to enemas and liquid glycerin suppositories, stimulant laxatives take a lot longer to stimulate a bowel movement — usually several hours, compared to 10 minutes. Most children on **PRE-M.O.P.** don't need stimulant laxatives. Constipation in these children typically isn't so advanced that you need to throw the proverbial kitchen sink at the problem.

The combination of osmotic laxatives and suppositories works very well for children who aren't toilet trained. However, some cases are particularly challenging. If your child remains constipated on the basic **PRE-M.O.P.** regimen, especially if your child is a superstar withholder who is struggling to potty train, it's reasonable to replace your osmotic laxative with a senna-based liquid or (if your child is older) Ex-Lax squares. You would still administer a glycerin suppository on any day your child doesn't poop spontaneously or doesn't fully evacuate.

In general, I don't recommend senna products as a replacement for rectal therapies, because they're generally not as effective at stimulating a bowel movement and because they take so much longer to work.

Suppositories and Enemas Are Safe, Too

A liquid glycerin suppository (LGS) is essentially a small version of a pediatric enema, which itself is half the size of an adult-sized enema. An LGS bulb is about the size of a large grape and contains pure liquid glycerin. A pediatric enema, about the size of a travel-size shampoo bottle, contains 2.25 ounces of phosphate combined with saline solution.

Though the key ingredient is different in LGS and store-bought enemas is different, both products stimulate evacuation of stool. Also, both invite opposition, even hostility, from physicians because of where they are inserted: in the rectum.

Worldwide, most doctors strongly favor oral treatments and object to those administered rectally — or consider them, at best, a very last resort to be used very sparingly. Our private Facebook support group includes members from Canada, Australia, the UK, Ireland, Germany, Romania, the Philippines, China, and numerous other countries, and most of these parents report that their pediatricians oppose enemas, though some members are able to find doctors amenable to **M.O.P.**

In general, persuading a physician to agree to rectal treatments is an uphill battle, and I applaud parents who are willing to follow their instincts and go it alone. I know it's not easy to defy your doctor's recommendations.

Below I discuss the common objections to liquid glycerin suppositories and enemas, all unsubstantiated or totally off base. You won't hear these concerns from physicians who are actually experienced with enemas. If your doctor raises these objections, you might ask whether the doctor has actually tried enema therapy with chronically constipated patients. I bet the answer will be "no." (Or "no way.")

Some of the objections below also pertain to solid glycerin suppositories, "bullets" of solid glycerin inserted rectally. In Pre-**M.O.**P. we use solid suppositories, or slivers of them, for children under age 2, because these children usually need less glycerin, and you can easily lower the dose with a solid suppository by slicing part of it off. For older children, liquid glycerin suppositories tend to be considerably more effective than solid suppositories, and they work more quickly, usually within 10 minutes. Solid suppositories can take up to several hours to stimulate a poop.

- **Dependence.** Physicians are fond of telling parents that repeated enemas or liquid glycerin suppositories will make children "dependent" on them to poop, and the child will end up with "lazy bowels." I've heard this, oh, about 2 million times. It's false. There is no science to back up this theory and no scientific reason to think it's true.

  In a chronically constipated child, the bowel is already not working normally. The rectum has become stretched by the pile-up, so it can't fully contract to expel stool, and the child doesn't sense the urge to poop. As I've explained, this becomes a vicious cycle: Because the child can't feel the urge, even more poop piles up, which stretches the rectum even more, further compromising the rectum's tone and sensation.

  Enemas and liquid glycerin suppositories clear out the rectum, giving it a chance to regain the sensation and propulsive power to fully empty. Once that happens, the child will no longer need enemas or suppositories. If your child poops only after an LGS or an enema, this is *not* a sign of dependence on enemas. It is a sign your child's rectum hasn't fully recovered.

  Dependence is something different. A patient with type 1 diabetes, for example, will always be dependent on insulin to live. Your child will not always rely on enemas or suppositories to poop, though it may take a while. In the meantime, if enemas are what it takes for your child to fully evacuate every day, what's wrong with that? Certainly, pooping with the help of a suppository or enema is a lot healthier than not pooping.

When a child who has overcome constipation experiences a recurrence and needs to start suppositories or enemas again, parents will sometimes say: "See, she's dependent on enemas to poop." But again, this scenario does not describe dependence. What's happened is the child has gotten back into the habit of withholding, for any number of reasons. To wean off rectal therapy again, the child will need to fully evacuate every day so the rectum can recover.

- **Anal tearing.** Your child's sphincter, the ring of muscle surrounding the anus, is safe. Think about it: An enema or suppository applicator is about the diameter of a pencil, whereas stool of a constipated child is often as wide as a jumbo sausage! The sphincter of a chronically constipated child is plenty accustomed to stretching wider than it does when you insert an enema or suppository tip. What's more, enema and LGS tips are made of flexible plastic, and you can add gobs of lubricant to help the tip slide in. Your child is a lot more likely to experience anal tearing and bloody stools from straining to poop while constipated than from pooping with the help of a suppository or enema.

- **Elimination of helpful gut flora.** Some parents ask me whether enemas or liquid glycerin suppositories wash out the intestinal bacteria that promote immunity and good digestion. There are not a ton of studies on the topic, but research on high-powered, pre-colonoscopy clean-outs suggests the effect is temporary.[4] I believe that for chronically constipated children, the benefits of stimulating full evacuation every day far outweighs any reduction in helpful gut bacteria. My patients who get daily enemas, even large-volume enemas, are no more prone to illness than other kids.

- **Electrolyte imbalance.** This concern pertains only to enemas, not liquid glycerin suppositories, because store-bought enema solution contains phosphate, an electrolyte. (Though the

4 Claire L. O'Brien et al. "Impact of Colonoscopy Bowel Preparation on Intestinal Microbiota," *PLOS One,* May 1, 2013, https://journals.plos.org/plosone/article?id=10.1371/journal.pone.0062815.

typical pediatric enema box is labeled "pediatric enema saline laxative," the active ingredient is phosphate.)

Electrolytes are chemicals in the blood that regulate nerve and muscle function, hydration, and blood pressure. Certainly, an electrolyte imbalance would be a serious problem, potentially damaging the kidneys and heart. But this simply does not happen in healthy children who are limited to one enema per day. (I would never recommend multiple daily phosphate enemas.)

How, in theory, could enemas cause an electrolyte imbalance? Well, when a child is given a phosphate enema, the colon absorbs this electrolyte. If the colon absorbs too much, the child could, theoretically, end up with a dangerously high phosphate level. But the human body does an excellent job of controlling our electrolyte levels! A child with normal kidney function will simply pee out the extra phosphate. If your child has kidney disease, use liquid glycerin suppositories rather than enemas.

I have never had a patient develop an electrolyte imbalance from enemas. Research shows that for healthy children who receive one enema per day, electrolyte imbalance is practically unheard of. Complications from enemas are so uncommon that a review of 39 studies conducted over 50 years found a total of just 15 cases of electrolyte imbalance in children ages 3 through 18[2]. Over 50 years! The vast majority involved children who had a chronic disease or were given more than one enema in a day.[5]

At any rate, liquid glycerin suppositories have zero chance of interfering with electrolyte levels because glycerin is not an electrolyte.

- **Emotional trauma.** No studies have considered whether enemas will "emotionally scar" a child, as numerous doctors have claimed, but I cannot find any basis for this concern. As far as I can tell, doctors who issue this warning to

5 J. Mendoza et al. Systematic review: the adverse effects of sodium phosphate enema, Alimentary Pharmacology and Therapeutics, 22 April 2007, https://onlinelibrary.wiley.com/doi/full/10.1111/j.1365-2036.2007.03354.x.

parents have no actual experience with enemas and little understanding of how distressing life can be for a child who is chronically constipated.

But that doesn't stop them from calling enemas "traumatic." In response to such a comment, one mom in our support group posted: "It is way more traumatic to poop in the middle of class and stink up a room full of kids who don't yet have a verbal filter. A quick, painless enema is much easier."

Compared to all that, enemas and liquid glycerin suppositories are a breeze!

As another mom posted: "My daughter likes how she feels afterward. Does she want enemas to end one day? Yes! But she is perfectly content because she has seen how getting them helps. And it has helped her to be comfortable pooping at school because she can feel the urge now."

For some children, enemas and suppositories can be uncomfortable at first, especially if the child's rectum is supremely stuffed with stool or the child feels tense. And it's only natural for parents to be apprehensive before administering a rectal therapy. But most kids, especially very young children, adjust quickly, and a variety of strategies can help older children relax. In Part 4, I offer tips on making the enema or LGS process easier and more comfortable both for the child and the adult administering the treatment.

Next, let's dive into the details of **PRE-M.O.P.**

Part 4

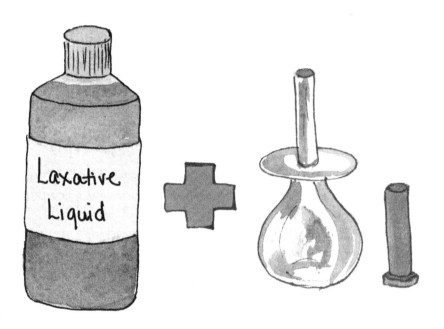

"We showed my son the enema ahead of time, told him the 'poo juice' would help his poop come out, and told him it might feel funny but won't hurt. The hardest part was getting him to lay down for the first few, but he quickly realized this didn't hurt and has since always been very cooperative."

Before I map out **PRE-M.O.P.**, I'll say it again: This program is intended for children who have not started toilet training or who are in the process of training and having trouble pooping on the potty. If your child has been toilet trained and continues to have accidents, **PRE-M.O.P.** is unlikely to suffice. You'll have more success with the full **M.O.P.** regimen. I know **PRE-M.O.P.** sounds easier, and it is, but a full-court press is in order.

PRE-M.O.P. Guidelines

PRE-M.O.P. involves far fewer choices than **M.O.P.** and just two components:

1) A daily osmotic laxative, taken either once a day or divided into two doses.

2) A suppository or enema in the evening if your child did not poop spontaneously during the day or if your child pooped but did not seem to have fully evacuated — for example, if you see just a smear of poop in the diaper and suspect the child is struggling to get more out. Children under age 2 use a solid glycerin suppository: those 2 and older use a liquid glycerin suppository or pediatric enema.

Here are guidelines for implementing the plan:

- Track the particulars. Each day, record the details of your child's treatment, such as the type of laxative given, the dose and time you gave it, and the child's output, including stool consistency and size and number of bowel movements. Part 5 includes a sample tracking calendar.

  You can download a full-size calendar under the **PRE-M.O.P.** section of our website, or you can create a spreadsheet or use any other paper or digital monitoring method. Whatever works!

- **Give the treatment a fair chance, but don't stick with products that aren't working.** I'm always astounded when a physician's response to a failed course of Miralax is: Take more Miralax! I'm not in favor of repeating a course of action that does not work.

It can take experimentation to find the laxative type and dose that hits the sweet spot: poop that's mushy but not too loose. Start by choosing one osmotic laxative, and stick with your choice for two weeks (unless, of course, your child has a bad reaction or rejects it because of the taste). During that time, experiment with the dose. You might also want to experiment with dividing the dose, giving half in the morning and half in the evening.

If, after two weeks, your child's stool is not considerably softer, try a different laxative, and adjust the dose and timing accordingly.

Some families on **M.O.P.** mix and match laxatives — for example, lactulose in the morning and magnesium citrate in the evening. With kids on **PRE-M.O.P.**, who haven't been constipated nearly as long, a single laxative usually does the job, but a combination is always an option.

Follow the same general rule of thumb for rectal therapy as you do for oral therapy: if you see no progress over two weeks, make a change. For example, adjust the dose of the solid suppository, or switch to an enema from a liquid glycerin suppository or vice versa.

- **If you aren't sure whether your child fully evacuated on a particular day, follow your instincts.** Remember, the general rule is to give a suppository or enema on any day the child does not poop at all or appears not to have fully evacuated. But how can you tell for sure whether the child emptied completely? You can't. You can only guess. Sometimes, it's obvious: you see a smear or tiny amount of stool, and the child's grimaces suggest the child is struggling to crank out more. In other cases, the child may not appear to be in distress but the output is meager. I usually err on the side of more aggressive treatment: you can't really go wrong giving a suppository to a chronically constipated child. But this is a gray area.

- **Don't worry if your child needs a suppository or enema several days in a row.** If you need to give your child rectal therapy every day for a few weeks, so be it. That just demonstrates how badly the child needs **PRE-M.O.P.**

Most constipated babies don't need consecutive enemas after the first week, but some do. Kids on **PRE-M.O.P.** who need daily enemas for longer than a week are usually 3-year-olds who have struggled with potty training and are considerably more clogged up than the typical constipated baby.

Parents who are new to rectally administered treatments are often surprised that a single suppository or enema won't fix the problem. But chronically constipated kids harbor more poop than you can imagine, and the holding habit can be deeply ingrained. **There's no overnight fix for chronic constipation.** The goal isn't just to clean out the rectum, which can fill right back up; it's to keep the rectum clear every single day so the child overcomes the withholding habit and the rectum shrinks back to size.

Sometimes, even the most savvy and proactive parents — those who've dealt with severe constipation in an older child and jumped on the earliest signs of constipation with a younger child — are astounded at how many suppositories a preschool-age child can need. One such mom emailed me in frustration after an x-ray showed her 4-year-old son — who has pee accidents, bedwetting, and a distended belly — was chock full of stool. She wrote:

"We thought because we jumped on his constipation so early — with Miralax and LGS shortly before he turned 3 — he'd be OK. How could he get this backed up when we used liquid glycerin suppositories almost daily?"

Constipation is sneaky. Even if you think you're completely on top of things, you can get behind. So don't worry about doing too many enemas or suppositories! The risk is in doing too few.

- **Plan to stick with osmotic laxatives until your child is at least a year past potty training and ideally through the first half of kindergarten.** Yes, kindergarten!

As I've mentioned, potty training is the number-one time for chronic constipation to develop (or worsen, if the child was constipated as a baby), and kindergarten poses additional challenges. Most kids are starting a new school, and even if the bathroom is contained within the classroom, students have to take more initiative to use it than they did in preschool. Their days are more structured, and their teachers, busy giving lessons on counting and the alphabet, are less likely to offer bathroom reminders.

The bottom line: go into **PRE-M.O.P.** expecting a long period of maintenance. I cannot count the number of patients who've been weaned off laxatives prematurely only to have a recurrence of constipation that leads to accidents and **M.O.P.**

You can try lowering the laxative dose about 6 months after potty training and see how things go. But if you notice your child's stools getting harder and/or larger, dial it back up and wait a few more months before you try lowering the dose again. It's important to keep a child's stools soft so she doesn't associate pooping with pain.

When you feel certain your child is out of the woods, ideally in kindergarten, try tapering laxatives to every other day for a few weeks and then twice a week for a few weeks and then stop.

Don't hesitate to start back up at the slightest hint of a recurrence.

- **Go back to suppositories or enemas any time your child doesn't poop.** Let's say your child stopped needing suppositories four months ago and then happens to go a day without pooping. Jump back on it! Don't wait an extra day to see if she'll poop. Make it happen now.

Often parents need to resume suppositories or enemas for a few days after a child has had a GI bug or other illness that makes pooping uncomfortable and restarts the withholding cycle. Plan for that, and keep suppositories in the house! Many pharmacies do not stock pediatric liquid or solid suppositories, so order a stash online.

Osmotic Laxative Options

I don't have strong feelings about which type of osmotic laxative a family should use, but you or your child might. What matters is keeping poop mushy, and there are many ways to accomplish this.

The world's most commonly prescribed osmotic laxative is PEG 3350, sold in the U.S. as Miralax or generic brands and sold as Movicol in Australia, New Zealand, and several European countries. I'm not going to rail against this laxative, as it has served many of my patients well and appears to be safe for the vast majority of children. However, I do take seriously the reports of psychiatric symptoms associated with PEG 3350, and I would never insist a parent use this laxative. I discuss these reports in the next section and include PEG 3350 last on the list of laxative options for **PRE-M.O.P.**

Keep in mind that you can switch osmotic laxatives at any time. So, if you notice your child is not improving on a particular laxative, has any kind of negative reaction, or appears not to like the taste, try a different one the next day. No weaning period is necessary.

Here is a rundown of osmotic laxatives appropriate for babies and toddlers.

- **Lactulose**

  This clear liquid (some brands have a red or green tint) is a manufactured sugar that contains two naturally occurring sugars, galactose and fructose. In many countries, lactulose can be purchased over the counter. In the United States it requires a prescription.

  Many children respond quite well to lactulose and prefer to swallow 2 teaspoons of this sweet, syrupy liquid than to drink a glass of water mixed with laxative powder. Lactulose is also quicker and easier for parents to administer, because there's no mixing required.

  Its potential side effects — diarrhea, nausea, gas — are the same as those linked with PEG 3350 and are generally mild if they occur. Some children have more gas or discomfort with lactulose than with PEG 3350, but others don't.

Dosing tips: For babies under 1 year, start with 2.5 ml twice a day or 5 ml daily. Toddlers may need more; 3-year-olds often start with 10 ml per day. Don't exceed 30 ml per day

• **Magnesium hydroxide, aka milk of magnesia**

Magnesium hydroxide is a naturally occurring mineral commonly sold as milk of magnesia, a liquid. It does not taste great! That's why chewable tablets, such as Pedialax Children's Chewable Saline Laxative Tablets, are popular. But, of course, babies can't chew tablets. Also, the tablets are costly, whereas milk of magnesia is quite inexpensive.

Dosing tips for magnesium hydroxide liquid: For a milk of magnesia solution with a typical concentration (the bottle will say 400 mg/5 ml), the typical recommended dose is 1 ml to 3 ml per kg of the child's weight — or 1 ml to 3 ml per half-pound of weight. So, a toddler who weighs 24 pounds (about 11 kg), would take 12 ml to 36 ml per day.

Dosing tips for magnesium hydroxide tablets: If your child can chew tablets, start with 1 to 3 chewable tablets per day, up to a maximum of 6 tablets.

• **Magnesium citrate**

Magnesium citrate is a popular option among parents who are not comfortable with Miralax. I recommend the liquid form, as powders may not contain enough magnesium citrate to have a laxative effect. (They're promoted as "anti-stress" beverages, not laxatives.)

Dosing tips: Dosages to treat chronic constipation are not well established, so you will need to experiment. For the liquid version, start with 150 to 300 ml. In general, the heavier the child, the greater the dose needed, but some smaller kids may need more, and some larger kids may need less.

• **PEG 3350 powder (Miralax and generic brands)**

PEG 3350 is a flavorless, odorless powder that you mix in water or other clear liquids. If your child prefers Miralax mixed in milk, that's fine. It won't compromise the effectiveness of the laxative — that's a myth! — though the powder doesn't mix as thoroughly in milk as it does in water.

Dosing tips: For a baby or toddler, start with 1/2 capful.

Dosing Stimulant Laxatives

As I mentioned in Part 3, most children on **PRE-M.O.P.** do very well on the combination of osmotic laxatives and suppositories and don't need stimulant laxatives. But if your child is a super-withholder and the regular **PRE-M.O.P.** regimen doesn't seem to be doing the job, add senna-based liquid, starting with 2 1/2 ml to 7 1/2 ml per day. Or, if your child is old enough to chew, start with 1 Ex-Lax square. You can make tiny increases, such as 1/4 or 1/2 a square. Sometimes a big jump can cause cramping.

Is Miralax Toxic for Children?

PEG 3350 is a fraught topic. Many physicians adamantly believe it's 100% safe, while many outraged parents report that their children were harmed by it.

What do I think?

I think Miralax and its generic equivalents do not cause problems in the vast majority of children. Among the 100+ published articles that have studied PEG 3350 in children, none have linked it to severe or harmful side effects, psychiatric or otherwise. These studies indicate PEG 3350 does not enter the child's bloodstream, has no effect on the body's balance of electrolytes, and just washes out the colon.

Nonetheless, a small minority of my patients and members of our private Facebook support group have reported worrisome, even alarming, symptoms upon giving their children Miralax, including rage, anxiety, and obsessive behavior. Thousands of consumers have reported these and other concerning side effects to the U.S. Food and Drug Administration's Adverse Event Reporting System.

I do not dismiss these reports and think it's possible that the reported symptoms were triggered by PEG 3350. At any rate, parents worried about PEG 3350 should not give it to their children. Period.

I treat Miralax like any medicine or food: if it causes problems, steer clear. Alternative laxatives, such as lactulose and magnesium hydroxide, work well and pose no safety concerns in recommended doses. I never insist parents give their children Miralax.

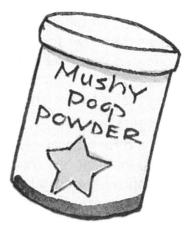

Why might PEG 3350 cause psychiatric symptoms in children? The answer, so far, is unknown. I suspect that in some children, the very real symptoms attributed to Miralax have other origins, and the discussion must be nuanced.

For example, here is a thoughtful post from a mom in our support group whose autistic son displayed frightening symptoms after taking Miralax at age 3 but tolerated it well when he was older:

> On Miralax he was manic-laughing in a distressed 'please help me' sort of way that was heart wrenching. It was definitely related to Miralax because if he skipped a day, his behavior returned to normal (for him). Because of this, we avoided Miralax for many years. However, when he was 9, we tentatively tried it again, and it's completely different now. No behavior changes at all.
>
> In retrospect, I believe that although the behavior changes were related to the Miralax, it might not have been directly caused by the Miralax. He is normally not very aware of the sensations going on in his body, but all of a sudden there's a massive change in the amount of movement in his GI, and he's not used to it, and the sensory experience could have just been too overwhelming. But things have changed as he's older, and he can tolerate the Miralax. Also, this time he's on **M.O.P.**, so things are moving and exiting more, which is much more comfortable for him than just forced leaking around a blockage.

A common argument against PEG 3350 is that it has not been approved by FDA for use in children. This is true, and in light of this fact, giving PEG 3350 to a child sounds irresponsible, if not outrageous. My own wife was alarmed, for this reason, when I gave Miralax to our children.

But I don't make much of the fact that Miralax isn't FDA-approved for kids. <u>Nearly 80 percent of hospitalized children</u> receive medications that are not approved for kids.[1] Once the FDA approves a drug for any indicated use, physicians may legally prescribe the drug for patients in other age groups. That's called off-label use, and it's common practice.

PEG 3350 was approved by the FDA for adults in 1999, is available over the counter, and is already taken by children all over the world every day. So, the manufacturer has no incentive to fund the complex, lengthy, and expensive process required to petition for the drug's approval in children. The fact that PEG 3350 is not FDA-approved for children does not mean it is unsafe for children.

Only a small number of drugs have been formally tested in children. Because PEG 3350 is actually one of them and because thousands of my patients have taken this drug without incident, I think it's fine if you want to use it.

And it's fine if you don't.

Suppository and Enema Options

For babies under age 1: Use a solid glycerin suppository labeled "for infants," or slice a children's solid glycerin suppository in half. Many pharmacies don't stock infant-sized suppositories.

For children 1 to 2: Use solid glycerin suppositories labeled "pediatric" or "children's."

For children 2+: Use liquid glycerin suppositories or pediatric enemas. Liquid suppositories work more quickly than solid

---

1 Children's Hospital of Philadelphia. "Most Children In US Hospitals Receive Medicines Off-label." ScienceDaily. www.sciencedaily.com/releases/2007/03/070305202847.htm

suppositories, and there's no chance the child will just "spit out" the suppository before it has a chance to stimulate a poop, as sometimes happens with solid suppositories.

For children on **PRE-M.O.P.**, I generally recommend LGS over pediatric enemas, which — despite being called pediatric "saline" enemas — actually contain phosphate (in saline solution) as their main ingredient. Some children experience a burning sensation in reaction to phosphate, and a baby or toddler won't be able to articulate that.

However, if your child is at least 2 and you're not seeing progress with liquid glycerin suppositories, try pediatric enemas. They are perfectly safe, and for many severely constipated children, are more effective than liquid glycerin suppositories. Most kids don't feel a burning sensation.

How to Give a Solid Glycerin Suppository

STEP 1: Remove the child's diaper, and wash your hands.

STEP 2: Show the suppository to the child, and explain what you're about to do and why.

Yes, do this even with an infant! It shows respect and demonstrates to your child that you are partners in this endeavor. This treatment isn't something you are doing to your child but rather with your child.

STEP 3: Put a dab of Vaseline or Aquaphor on the child's anus.

STEP 4: Place your child in any of three positions:

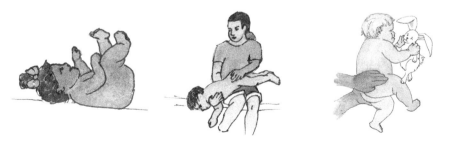

STEP 5: Insert the suppository into the rectum with your finger, pushing it past the sphincter (about $1/2$ to 1 inch in).

STEP 6: Hold your child's buttocks together for a few seconds.

This can help keep the suppository in place, but if a child is extremely backed up, the suppository may be crowded out and just pop out. If that happens, try again the next day. The laxative alone may clear out enough stool for you to get the suppository into place.

STEP 7: Put the child's diaper back on, and wash your hands.

How to Give a Liquid Glycerin Suppository or Enema

What you need: LGS or enema (squeeze bottle, lubricated tip) and lubricant such as Vaseline, K-Y jelly, or Aquaphor. Experiment and see which lubricant works best for you and your child.

Wash your hands before you remove the enema from the box. Then follow these steps.

STEP 1: Show your child the bottle, applicator, lubricated tip, and extra lubrication.
Explain what you're about to do, and briefly review why, even if your child is too young to fully understand what you're staying. It's important to convey that the two of you are in this together.

If your child seems apprehensive, mention that the extra lubrication will help the tip slide in easily.

STEP 2: Place a towel on the floor or bed, and position your child on the left side, knees bent toward the chest, aiming for the belly button. Because of the colon's anatomy, lying on the left side helps the emptying process and is more comfortable for the child. However, with young children, some parents find it easier if the child is positioned on her back with knees bent or positioned on her knees, facedown, with her bottom up. Or, try any of the other positions listed in the box titled "5 Positions for Your Child to Try."

STEP 3: Rub lubricant on the applicator, on your child's anus, and on the surrounding skin, to reduce possible irritation from overspray of stool.

Gently insert the applicator into the child's bottom, making sure it gets past the sphincter.

You'll know you're in when you pass the point of resistance. If your child seems tense, encourage your child to take deep breaths, like blowing out birthday candles.

STEP 4: Squeeze the bulb or bottle slowly and steadily until you have emptied as much as directed by your doctor or the package. Enema companies recommend using half a bottle of the pediatric enema for children ages 2 to 5 (yes, you can use the rest the next day). Liquid glycerin suppositories are smaller, so you use all the fluid.

Enema bottles have a one-way valve, so you can release and squeeze again to make sure you've emptied most of the liquid. It's not necessary to empty the entire contents, as enemas and liquid glycerin suppositories contain more liquid than is needed to stimulate a bowel movement.

In some children who are extremely clogged, inserting the liquid stretches the rectum to the point of pain. If this happens, stop and encourage your child to poop.

The discomfort should diminish with each day, as the rectum empties.

STEP 5: When nearly all the solution has been flushed into your child's rectum, remove the applicator, and put on a fresh diaper. Your child will likely poop within 20 minutes, though it usually happens within a few minutes.

5 Positions for Your Child to Try

There's no single best way to position a child for an enema or liquid glycerin suppositories. Different kids have different preferences. When I asked members of our support group to describe the positions their kids prefer, the answers were all over the map! Here are a few of the responses:

- "On his back with one of us holding his legs towards his chest."
- "Lying on her left side, mainly because she is watching the iPad while we do it."
- "Lying on her back with me holding his knees to her chest. He won't do it any other way."
- "She lies across my lap, with her bottom in the air, while clutching her favorite toy."
- "On her knees, chest down, bum up."

Try them all and see which your child prefers!

Part 5

Tracking Your Child on PRE- M.O.P.

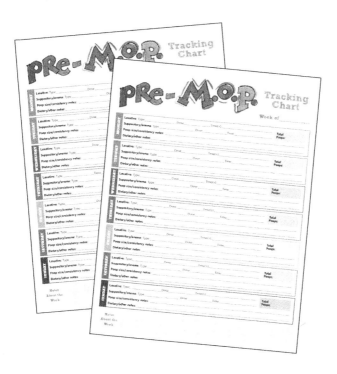

"Oh man. I tracked EVERYTHING. How long he held the enema, what his poop looked like afterward, the type and dose of laxative. Tracking helped me realize Miralax made my son feel bloated and gassy, so we switched to magnesium citrate. Overall, tracking made me feel in control, like we had a plan."

Tracking a child's progress on **PRE-M.O.P.** will alert you to patterns and help you make decisions along the way.

For example, your notes may prompt you to try a different laxative or adjust the dose until you find that happy medium: poop that's mushy but not runny.

One mom who was giving her daughter Ex-Lax discovered, via her tracking calendar, that a single square wasn't producing much poop. "I upped it to 1 1/4 squares and then 1 3/4 square and it still wasn't enough," she posted. "When we got to 2 squares, it produced a morning poop that isn't too soft or messy. She takes it at dinner, because she had gas pain if she takes it in the morning."

" Tracking made me feel in control, like we had a plan."

It is important to re-evaluate your child's overall progress on **PRE-M.O.P.** every week. If you see no improvement, make a change.

Sometimes parents will say, "We did **M.O.P.** for 6 months, and it didn't work." Yet they never adjusted the regimen! With **M.O.P.**, we advise making a change after 30 days without progress; with **PRE-M.O.P.**, tweak the regimen after a week without improvement.

If your child is a baby, I suggest tracking your child's pooping patterns for about a month after she stops showing signs of constipation. Then, resume tracking a week before you start potty training, to make triple sure your child is still pooping a pile of mush every day. Don't start potty training a constipated child!

Once you start toilet training, switch from the **PRE-M.O.P.** chart to one of the two potty-training charts in Part 6. These provide space to track peeing, too. Some kids with a history of holding poop also hold pee, behavior that — as I explain in Part 6— exacerbates constipation symptoms.

PRe-M.O.P. Tracking Chart

Week of _____

MONDAY
Laxative: Type_____ Dose_____ Time(s)_____
Suppository/enema: Type_____ Dose_____ Time(s)_____
Poop size/consistency notes: _____ Dose_____ Time_____
Dietary/other notes:_____
Total Poops:

TUESDAY
Laxative: Type_____ Dose_____ Time(s)_____
Suppository/enema: Type_____ Dose_____ Time(s)_____
Poop size/consistency notes: _____ Dose_____ Time_____
Dietary/other notes:_____
Total Poops:

WEDNESDAY
Laxative: Type_____ Dose_____ Time(s)_____
Suppository/enema: Type_____ Dose_____ Time(s)_____
Poop size/consistency notes: _____ Dose_____ Time_____
Dietary/other notes:_____
Total Poops:

THURSDAY
Laxative: Type_____ Dose_____ Time(s)_____
Suppository/enema: Type_____ Dose_____ Time(s)_____
Poop size/consistency notes: _____ Dose_____ Time_____
Dietary/other notes:_____
Total Poops:

FRIDAY
Laxative: Type_____ Dose_____ Time(s)_____
Suppository/enema: Type_____ Dose_____ Time(s)_____
Poop size/consistency notes: _____ Dose_____ Time_____
Dietary/other notes:_____
Total Poops:

SATURDAY
Laxative: Type_____ Dose_____ Time(s)_____
Suppository/enema: Type_____ Dose_____ Time(s)_____
Poop size/consistency notes: _____ Dose_____ Time_____
Dietary/other notes:_____
Total Poops:

SUNDAY
Laxative: Type_____ Dose_____ Time(s)_____
Suppository/enema: Type_____ Dose_____ Time(s)_____
Poop size/consistency notes: _____ Dose_____ Time_____
Dietary/other notes:_____
Total Poops:

Notes
About the
Week

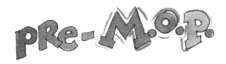

Sample #1

This child took two 5-ml doses of lactulose, pooped soft snakes, and pooped after the LGS. "No SP" means "no spontaneous poop."

MONDAY

Laxative: Type _Lactulose_   Dose _5 ml x 2_   Time(s) _8 am / 6pm_

Suppository/enema: Type _LGS_   Dose _____   Time _6:15 pm_

Poop size/consistency notes: _Good output - soft snakes_

Dietary/other notes: _still no SP_

Total Poops: _1_

Sample #2

This child strained to produce a few pellets at 11 a.m. so the parent decided that was not a full evacuation (hence "1.5" total poops) and gave a whole solid suppository (noted as "SS," with "full" dose) at 5 p.m. which was followed 2 hours later by a medium-size pile.

TUESDAY

Laxative: Type _Miralax_   Dose _1/2 cap_   Time(s) _7 am_

Suppository/enema: Type _SS_   Dose _full_   Time _5 pm_

Poop size/consistency notes: _a few pellets @ 11 am / med. pile @ 7 pm_

Dietary/other notes: _strained to poop in am_

Total Poops: _1.5_

Sample #3

This child took a.m. and p.m. doses of milk of magnesia (aka "MoM"), pooping a hard log at 9 a.m. and a meager watery poop at 6 p.m.

SATURDAY

Laxative: Type _MoM_ Dose _15 ml x 2_ Time(s) _6:30 am / 4 pm_	**Total Poops:** 2
Suppository/enema: Type _enema_ Dose _____ Time _6:30 pm_	
Poop size/consistency notes: _hard log 9 am / watery poop 6 pm_	
Dietary/other notes: _expected more output after enema_	

Sample #4

Two weeks of eliminating dairy didn't seem to help this child. She did not poop on her own 6 out of 7 days and was given LGS on those days. Her parent noted she seems more comfortable than before starting suppositories.

Notes About the Week

2nd week of no dairy - made no diff.

did LGS 6 days

Only one SP. Poops still mostly hard.

she seems more comfortable than b/4 LGS

Part 6

Toilet Training and Beyond: The Surveillance Years

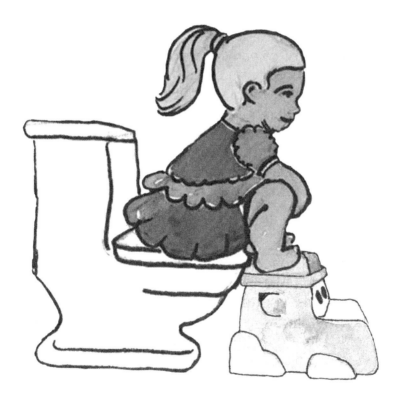

"The world doesn't actually implode if your child starts school in nappies!"

Our culture gets potty training exactly wrong. In books and articles, the emphasis is inevitably on completing the process at warp speed. Potty train in 3 days! Potty train your kiddo ASAP! In a weekend! In an afternoon! Potty train before age 2! Avoid diapers and train from birth!

And if you don't have the time or inclination to do the job yourself? Just send your kid to potty boot camp or hire a private coach.

Whatever it takes, get this sucker done!

The arguments in favor of early and speedy training are all over the map. Among the most popular: If you don't hurry up, that "window of opportunity" will slam shut, and you'll be left with a potty "refuser" who will require diapers in kindergarten. Another common argument is that some Asian and African cultures don't use diapers, so why should we? Parents who drag out potty training until age 3, these folks argue, are just coddling their children and clogging our landfills.

Preschools tend offer a more practical argument: they just don't have enough staff to change diapers.

Some potty-training coaches prey on the insecurities we all have as parents, our fears that we won't measure up. "Be wary of well-meaning friends who tell you that your child is too young" to potty train, one author asserts, because these so-called friends "have an emotional investment in your failure." If you follow this author's plan and finish the job by the time your child is age 2 $\frac{1}{2}$, she assures readers, "You are going to have awesome bragging rights."

Geez, parenting is not a competitive sport! And what kind of "friends" have an emotional investment in your failure, anyway?

As the parent of a chronically constipated child, you'll need a stiff spine. You'll have to resist the pressure to toilet train on someone else's schedule, for someone else's reasons, and with someone else's speed-training methods. You may even need to find a different preschool, because the stakes are too high to risk training your child before she's ready.

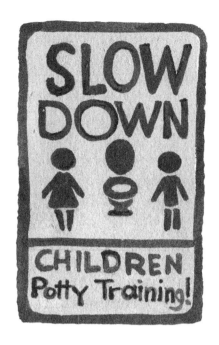

The fact is, any child who struggled with constipation as a baby or toddler will be at high risk for a recurrence during the toilet-training process and for developing enuresis and/or encopresis down the road. It's important to place your child in an environment where nobody — not your child and not you — feels pressure to leave diapers behind.

Helping your child avoid bedwetting as a 4th grader is more important than having "awesome bragging rights" now. That's obvious. But when you're out in the real world, at the park or a birthday party or any place where parents are judging other people's parenting, this fact is easy to forget.

No matter what others say, getting the job done right is far more important than getting it done quickly. This is a lesson **M.O.P.** parents have learned well. As one mom in our support group posted:

> *Having a child on **M.O.P.** has really helped me to get over the whole social stigma aspect. I don't feel any pressure to push my younger two to learn because a) the older they are when they decide to quit nappies, the better they'll be at listening to and responding to their bodies, and b) the world doesn't actually implode if your child starts school in nappies!*

What many preschools don't realize is that toilet training, unlike, say, learning to ride a bike, is not a skill that gets "locked in" with a bit of practice. Or tied up in a knot that will never unravel. Acing a 3-day boot camp does not *in any way* guarantee a child will in the future heed her body's signals to use the toilet.

For most of us, learning to pee and poop on the potty is easy; what's difficult is acting on, rather than overriding, our body's urges to pee and poop — every day, every time the urge strikes. I have numerous patients who were "successfully" toilet trained before age 2 only to start having accidents in kindergarten, after their withholding habit went unnoticed for years.

The most important skill kids must master is not pooping in the toilet or avoiding accidents. It is peeing and pooping in a timely manner. But this benchmark is hard for adults to gauge. You can count the number of accidents a child has had, and believe me, preschools do! One mom in our support group was told her daughter had had the most accidents "in the history of the school." But you can't count how many times a child has squeezed her sphincter to override the brain's signal to empty the rectum. The best you can do is delay toilet training until your child seems sufficiently mature and to watch like a hawk for signs of constipation and pee holding.

Forget bragging rights. When it comes to potty training your child, the *only* two considerations should be: 1.) Has your child overcome constipation? and 2.) Is your child sufficiently mature?

In this part I offer guidelines for successfully potty training a child with a history of constipation. And by "success," I don't mean getting your child out of diapers. I mean setting your child up for a lifetime of healthy toileting habits.

Most of this advice applies to children without a history of constipation, but it's all the more critical for children who've been through **PRE-M.O.P.**

8 Rules for Potty Training Kids with a History of Constipation

 Watch closely for any signs that constipation has returned.

Don't even think about toilet training until your child has been free of all signs of constipation for several months. This means your child poops a pile of mush *every single day*, and you can barely remember a time when she didn't.

To ensure your child maintains this super pooping, continue with the osmotic laxative throughout toilet training and at least one year beyond, ideally through the beginning of kindergarten. Continue to use a liquid glycerin suppository in the evening if your child didn't spontaneously poop during the day. Even if you haven't used an LGS in many months, be prepared to start up again during potty training.

No matter how well potty training seems to be going, keep a close watch for the signs of constipation. After all you've been through, you cannot afford to take your eye off the ball!

If your child attends preschool, ask the teacher for a daily report on whether, and how many times, your child pooped or peed. Ask your child, too, and assess whether the reports match.

The two charts in this section can help you look for the red flags. It's easy to forget the last time your child pooped or peed; a few notes can help. Don't stress yourself out logging every detail for months. A week may provide insight.

As a reminder, here, in no particular order, are telltale signs of constipation in children who are toilet training.

- Extra-large stools
- Pellet-shaped stools
- Reluctance to poop on the toilet
- Hiding to poop

- Pooping less often than once a day
- Pooping more often than once a day
- Underwear "skid marks" or itchy bottom
- Belly pain
- Mad dashes to the toilet
- Incessant peeing
- Pee accidents
- Poop accidents
- Bedwetting at age 4 or older

Download the "How's Your Poop?" chart from our website and post it on the bathroom wall.[1] Teach your child to identify her poops in the pictures and peer into the toilet bowl yourself. You'll get used to it!

Wait until your child is ready to toilet train.

Again, "ready" does not mean that your preschool is ready or that you are ready. It means that in addition to having overcome constipation, your child demonstrates the maturity to listen to her body's signals, even when she's engrossed in finger painting.

Ideally, wait until your child:

- Can dress and undress without help.
- Shows interest in using the toilet.
- Notices when she has a wet or dirty diaper.
- Tells you when she needs to pee or poop.

Most children meet these benchmarks around age 3, but that is not a hard-and-fast rule.

If you feel swayed by the "window of opportunity" argument or feel compelled to justify your "late" training to a friend or a preschool, read a study conducted at my clinic. The results

---

1 https://www.bedwettingandaccidents.com/downloads-in-english

> *"My 11-year-old son has been constipated since he was a baby. I have no doubt that this problem could have been prevented by not trying to potty train him so early, at 2, and by taking more seriously his giant poops and his purposeful poop holding."*

clearly demonstrate that early training is a risky proposition.[2]

We studied 112 children ages 3 to 10 and found that those trained before age 2 had *triple* the risk of developing constipation and daytime enuresis compared to children who trained between ages 2 and 3.

Of course, many children who trained early are lucky enough to emerge unscathed. You probably know kids like this and have forced a smile as their parents exercised those "bragging rights." But in fact, the odds aren't terrific for these kids: **In our study, 60% of children toilet trained before age 2 presented with daytime enuresis.**

An important note: our results do not suggest that training between ages 2 and 3 is better than training at age 3 or later — just that training between ages 2 and 3 is better than training earlier. In my experience, the closer kids are to age 3, the less likely they are to struggle.

To meet preschool potty deadlines, many parents start training their children between 18 months and 2 years. Understandably, they want to avoid the panic that strikes when preschool starts in 3 weeks and their child still

> *"I wish I had been more patient with my child and worried less what other people thought."*

won't venture near the toilet. Parents figure: *If we start early, we won't have to rush, and my child won't feel pressure.*

2   Steve Hodges, et al., "The association of age of toilet training and dysfunctional voiding," *Research and Reports in Urology,* 3 October 2014 Volume 2014:6, pp 127-130. https://doi.org/10.2147/RRU.S66839.

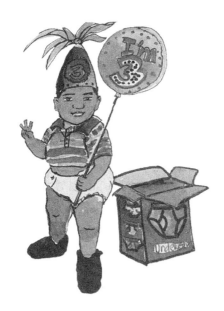

Most children are ready to potty train around age 3, not age 2.

All that sounds logical. The problem is, the extra time won't help a child who isn't ready. It's like trying to teach a 1st-grader to do long division so the child can get a jump on the skills required in 5th-grade. Of course, there will always be prodigies to whom the rules don't apply, whether you're talking about potty training or math. But in general, teaching children a new skill before they are developmentally ready will be frustrating at best and at worst will backfire big time.

Potty-training deadlines generate much anxiety in parents and children and are responsible for countless cases of toileting dysfunction. If you can't find a satisfactory preschool without an age-3 mandate, delay training until your child is as close to age 3 as possible. Kids around age 3 who aren't constipated can often learn toilet training within a week. **Giving a child more time to mature is far more helpful than giving a child more time to learn toileting.**

What about those 4-year-olds who can't seem to graduate from diapers?

Parents whose preschoolers struggle to train are often blamed for waiting too long and missing that legendary window of opportunity. But as our data shows, the problem is not slacker parenting; it's constipation. When a 4-year-old "refuses" to poop on the toilet, it's because the child is constipated and pooping hurts, not because the child is hellbent on exercising her free will and defying you.

Two Ways to Encourage a Reluctant Child to Poop on the Potty

What if you're sure your child is both mature enough to use the toilet and no longer constipated — but the child still insists on pooping in a diaper?

I have two approaches to suggest.

The Hole-in-the-Diaper Method

This strategy is borrowed from *The Ins and Outs of Poop* by Thomas DuHamel and Kevin Brockschmidt. Some parents I know swear by it. You take each of the following steps for about three days before encouraging your child to move on to the next step. If your child balks during any step, don't push it. Just remain where the child feels comfortable.

- **STEP 1: Ask your child to poop in the bathroom.**
  Assure the child that pooping in a diaper or pull-up is absolutely fine! All you're suggesting is the child do the deed in the bathroom. If all goes well, move on to the next Step 2.

- **STEP 2: Ask your child to poop in a pull-up *while sitting on the toilet*.**
  Again, assure your child: pull-ups are cool! No issue there! You're just going to try unloading in the seated position, on the potty. Success? Move on to Step 3.

- **STEP 3: Cut a hole in the pull-up, and ask your child to poop while wearing the cut-out diaper.**
  Yeah, this sounds weird! But some kids are willing to poop on the toilet if they're allowed to maintain the security of their beloved pull-up.

- **STEP 4: Make the diaper hole much bigger, and repeat Step 3.**
  After a few days of pooping through the hole, your child may willingly transition to pooping through a giant hole — a hole so big that basically the kid is wearing a shredded diaper belt.

- **STEP 5**: Encourage your child to poop right into the potty, without the diaper belt.
  With confidence gained from steps 1 through 4, your child may feel ready to go for it! But if not, don't push it. Your child will come around eventually, as long as constipation remains resolved.

The Ex-Lax Method

Sometimes kids with a history of ignoring their bodies' urges just need some nudging — not from you, but from their body — to get over the hump.

For these kids, a few days of stimulating a bowel movement with Ex-Lax can help. Once a child's rectum has been fully cleaned out and has regained sensation, it's hard for the child to override the body's signal to poop. You can capitalize on this by artificially stimulating the bowel movement with a few squares of Ex-Lax or a couple doses of senna-based liquid.

In this case, the laxative is not being used to clean out the rectum — I am assuming your child is already cleaned out — but rather to demonstrate to the child that pooping no longer hurts. Once the child has a few of these stimulated bowel movements and realizes pooping is no longer a strain, the child may be cool with the whole pooping thing. If your child remains reluctant to poop on the toilet, back off. You definitely don't want to encourage the holding habit.

Let your child lead the way

When it comes to potty training, your child is boss!

This is tough for some parents to accept, but it's reality. You can't compel a child to poop or pee in the toilet any more than you can compel her to sleep, so let go of all your plans and expectations. Pressuring your child or micromanaging the process will backfire eventually, if not immediately. Step aside and allow your child to own this milestone.

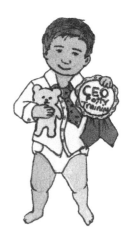

Some forms of pressure are overt. For example: "If you're not potty trained by September, they won't let you into preschool!" Or: "You're old enough to be out of diapers by now!" These are words no parent should ever utter. **Any sort of punishment, "consequence," or display of disappointment should never play a role in the potty-training process.**

But you can sabotage toilet training with more subtle forms of pressure, such as excessive rewards or praise. For example: offering extra screen time, a "certificate of achievement," or a princess party for staying dry in underwear. Or: "Yay! You're such a big boy! You didn't have any accidents!"

These approaches may prompt your child to hold pee or poop in order to please you or earn a reward. **The message you're sending is: Staying dry is really important! But the message you want to send is: Use the toilet when your body tells you it's time!**

Letting your child be CEO of the potty-training enterprise doesn't mean you should disappear from the scene. You're the support staff. Here are some gentle ways to help your child master toilet training.

- **Tell your child she gets to set the timeline.** For instance: "Let me know when you feel ready to try using the potty" and "You get to decide when you want to wear underwear instead of a diaper."

- **Lead by example.** Invite your child to join you in the bathroom, and explain what's what. Say something like, "I got that feeling in my body that it was time to pee, so I went to the toilet right away."

- **Explain why it's important to poop daily and pee often.** Everyone loves the book *Everybody Poops*, but this fun potty-training classic doesn't explain *why* everybody poops. Preschoolers are capable of understanding that if you don't let poop out, it piles up inside and can give you a stomach ache. They can understand that the bladder ("a bag that holds your pee") can "get upset" if pee stays in too long. Our book *Jane and the Giant Poop* is a helpful and fun teaching tool.

- **Help your child recognize — and act on — the urge to pee or poop.**

  If you notice your child doing the potty dance, that elaborate number involving squirming, curtseying, or crotch grabbing, say, "I notice you're squeezing your legs together. This means you have to go pee, so let's walk to the bathroom."

- **Away from home, point out where the toilet is** — at the supermarket, the park, or a friend's house. Children who avoid public restrooms are more prone to withholding. It's important to get kids peeing and pooping away from home from the get-go. Carry a foldable, portable potty seat with you, so you can easily place it on any toilet.

- **Keep a potty in the car.** Make it super easy for your child to pee or poop as soon as the urge strikes!

- **Offer periodic reminders to use the toilet.** Yes, I know I said your child is boss. But you should still explain that growing children need to pee every 2 hours and that it's important to sit and try to poop after breakfast and dinner. Children who are newly potty trained need a lot of reminders and follow-up, no matter how well they seem to have grasped the concept.

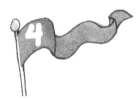 Watch closely for pee holding

Few kids want to interrupt their lives to use the toilet, so during the potty-training process, many children not only withhold poop but also withhold pee. Parents don't usually notice this behavior. They're too busy celebrating the fact that they don't have to change diapers.

If you've been focused all this time on your child's pooping problems, peeing issues may not even be on your radar. But they should be, because holding pee makes constipation symptoms far worse.

You might have heard that holding pee is a good thing, that it helps stretch the bladder so kids can hold more urine. Those Las Vegas teachers I mentioned in the introduction — the ones who told parents their children were "wasting valuable teaching time on bathroom breaks" — even advised parents to have their 1st-graders "practice to increase bladder endurance" so these kids would be able to limit bathroom trips to once or twice during the school day. Their instructions to parents: "Have him/her wait 15 minutes from their first urge and increase the wait time by 5 minutes per day over the course of two weeks until your child is able [to] hold their urine for two hours at a time."

This is some bad advice! Emptying every 2 to 3 hours, is what leads to healthy bladder growth. Holding urine actually serves to shrink bladder capacity and aggravate the bladder, setting a child up for enuresis, urinary tract infections, and other problems.

How so? Well, the bladder is basically a bag designed to hold pee. This bag empties through an outlet known as the bladder neck, which stays closed except when you're peeing. The bladder neck remains closed without any effort on your part.

But the bladder is not just a bag; it's a muscular bag that can stretch from about 2 inches in diameter to about 6 inches, depending on how much urine it's holding. When the bladder is not storing urine, it's squeezing to empty urine through the bladder neck, via a tube called the urethra. Every time you feel the urge to pee, you're feeling your bladder begin to squeeze and your bladder neck open up a bit.

Now, we all have the power, at least temporarily, to override this urge, by squeezing the external urethral sphincter, a band of muscle that wraps around the urethra and controls urine flow. Squeezing this sphincter tells the spinal cord to stop the bladder contraction. Most adults do this only when we need to, like when we're in the car or at the movies.

The problem is, each time you squeeze your sphincter to override your bladder's signal, you create resistance that strains your bladder. What happens when muscles go up against resistance? Exactly what happens when you train your biceps at the gym: they get thicker and stronger. Essentially the sphincter is engaged in a tug-of-war against the bladder: The bladder is trying to empty, while the sphincter is trying to hold in the urine. When the sphincter wins, you are dry; when the bladder wins, you're wet.

The sphincter always starts off stronger. That's the only way anyone could stay dry. Holding pee occasionally doesn't lead to any appreciable change in the bladder muscle. But when a child delays peeing multiple times a day over months and years, the bladder wall becomes thicker and more muscular. Eventually, the bladder capacity decreases, and the bladder contracts more forcefully.

I don't think this is what the Las Vegas teachers had in mind!

To make matters worse, the sensation mechanism of a thick-walled bladder goes haywire. Your child may get the signal that her bladder is full when it's only partially full. What's more, her bladder may start to have frequent, spontaneous, forceful contractions, like hiccups. This is what's happening when your child makes a mad dash to the bathroom. These sprints are the first sign of the chronic holding problem.

Eventually the bladder gets so strong and irritable that it empties without any input from the child, and the sphincter can't stop the emptying. That's enuresis.

Just imagine how much worse things are when a child's bladder is already irritable from having being squished by a stool-stuffed rectum!

Here's how to promote a healthy cycle of filling and emptying:

- **Establish a pee schedule that fits naturally into the day.**

  To prevent holding, it's best for newly trained children to pee even before they feel the urge. Encourage your child to pee before bed, first thing in the morning, and about every 2 hours during the day.

  When it has been 2 hours since your child peed or when you see your child do the potty dance, don't ask, "Do you need to go potty?" Children always say no! Instead, try something like: "It's time to go to the bathroom now, so your bladder can stay healthy and grow!"

- **Give your child plenty of fluids to stimulate emptying.**

  Let your child pick out a special cup or water bottle to take with him wherever he goes, like to the store, on playdates, and to preschool. He should drink a few ounces of fluid every few hours so his bladder doesn't fill too quickly (rapid filling can cause overactivity) or stay empty for extended periods of time. A bladder is happiest when it is cycling.

- **Encourage your child to relax on the potty and "let it all out."**

  Many kids empty just enough urine to relieve the urge, proclaiming, "All done!" before darting off to play. Watch your child as she pees. Does she hold her breath? Is her face turning red? Do her belly muscles seem tight? Kids with a history of straining to poop sometimes think they need to push to pee. If you notice your child straining, encourage her to breathe deeply and slowly and to keep her belly soft when she pees.

  I like to have kids sit for about 5 minutes at each attempt at peeing. Many kids respond better to an egg timer than to a parent. Keep your child's favorite books, puzzles, or toys by the toilet, and encourage her to stay busy while she waits for more pee to exit.

- **Teach your son to pee while seated and your daughter to pee with her legs spread.**

  Boys of potty-training age tend to relax and empty more fully when they are seated. Standing, on the other hand, prompts them to jut the pelvis forward, to get close enough to the toilet bowl. As a result, they squeeze their butt and pelvic floor muscles.

  As for girls, peeing with their legs spread ensures the urine flows from the bladder into the toilet without pooling in the vagina. When the vaginal skin stays wet, the child is more susceptible to urinary tract infections (which are, in the first place, triggered by constipation).

Provide a tall stool for pooping

The advent of the flush toilet made life easier but, ironically, did not make pooping easier. Quite the opposite.

That's because **human beings were designed to squat while pooping.**

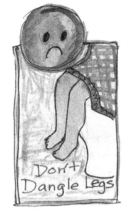

Don't Dangle Legs

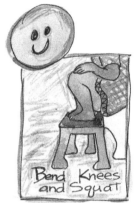

Bend Knees and Squat

You'd think sitting upright on a toilet would make gravity work in your favor, giving poop a straight shot downward. But human plumbing is not what it seems. In reality, when you stand, your rectum is bent, a position that helps keep poop safely inside. When you squat, the rectum straightens, and poop exits without effort on your part.

Anyone who has camped in the woods knows how easily you poop when you use nature's facilities. Sitting upright on the toilet, by contrast, is like trying to poop uphill.

Research even demonstrates that pooping in a squat is easier. In an Israeli study, subjects took 2 minutes and 10 seconds to poop when seated on a standard toilet: With their feet planted on a stool, they pooped in just 51 seconds.[3]

Yet the world's toilets are getting taller, placing us further and further away from a squat position. Standard toilets, 14 or 15 inches from floor to rim, have given way to 17-inch or even 19-inch "comfort height toilets." Companies boast that taller toilets "make sitting down and standing up easier for most adults, ensuring extra comfort."

3 Dov Sikirov. "Comparison of Straining During Defecation in Three Positions: Results and Implications for Human Health." *Digestive Diseases and Sciences*, 48 (7), July 2003: 1201–1205, https://www.ncbi.nlm.nih.gov/pubmed/12870773.

But for kids, what these taller toilets ensure is more pooping problems! (They make pooping harder for adults, too, which is why the Squatty Potty has become such a phenomenon.)

To poop easily and comfortably, kids need an extra-tall stool, like the children's version of the Squatty Potty or any similar stool.

The combination of a stool and kid-sized toilet seat also helps children relax their inner thighs and potty muscles. Think about it: Do you fully relax your body when you're sitting on a barstool without a footrest? Nope!

With their feet dangling, kids instinctively clench their inner thighs and pelvic floor muscles to keep from falling in. We can't see kids clenching, and they may not know they're doing it, but I assure you, they are.

A Japanese study that recorded the abdominal pressure of volunteers while they pooped found that the subjects strained less in the squatting position.[4] You can bet that young children, whose feet don't even reach the floor, strain even more than adults when perched on a toilet.

Depending on your child's size, you might also have your child sit on a potty seat. The seat will keep your child from falling into the toilet or worrying about it.

Never shame or blame your child for accidents.

It's natural for children to have accidents when they're learning to use the toilet. But if your child continues to have accidents after a month or so of training, chances are the child was not ready to train and/or is still constipated. Either way, your child is not responsible for these accidents, in the same way she is not responsible when she has hiccups or the flu. Showing disappointment or having your child clean up the mess as a "natural consequence" suggests otherwise, and that's unfair.

4 Ryuji Sakakibara. "Influence of Body Position on Defecation in Humans." *Lower Urinary Tract Symptoms*. 13 April 2010. https://onlinelibrary.wiley.com/doi/abs/10.111 1/j.1757-5672.2009.00057.

Given all you now know about recognizing and treating constipation, your child is unlikely to get to that point. By tracking your child's daily pooping, you'll probably notice signs and start aggressive treatment well before your child develops enuresis or encopresis. But sometimes, constipation can sneak up on you, and a child will have accidents despite numerous precautions.

If your child has accidents at preschool, explain to the school that your child has a history of chronic constipation and that accidents are symptoms of this medical condition, *not* a sign of willful behavior or a failure to understand potty training. Many preschool directors and teachers do not understand this and heap shame and blame upon 3- and 4-year-olds who have accidents. Our book *Bedwetting and Accidents Are Not Your Fault* can help kids feel better about having accidents.

 Do not attempt "night time" potty training.

In a potty-training book on my shelf, one author tells parents: "Becoming dry at night requires a devoted effort on your part. Don't shirk your parental responsibilities at this final hurdle!"

This is false! You cannot "train" a child to achieve dryness overnight any more than you can train a baby to crawl. Night-time potty training is just not a thing.

Overnight dryness happens naturally, typically by age 4. You cannot speed up the process by withholding pull-ups, limiting fluids before bed, or waking your child overnight to pee.

Despite what you may have heard, diapers are not a "crutch" that delays a child's ability or reduces her motivation to stay dry at night.

A child who is not constipated and has a healthy, stable bladder will easily make it through the night without peeing, even if he drinks a glass of water right before bed. Sure, a child who guzzles a gallon of water minutes before hitting the pillow may need to pee overnight, but withholding fluids after dinnertime is not a winning strategy.

If a child is wetting the bed at age 4 or beyond, I recommend treatment with **M.O.P.** Most doctors will tell you to wait until your child is at least 7, but I strongly disagree with that advice. Waiting around for a child to outgrow bedwetting serves no one.

 ## Don't ever stop asking your kids how often they poop.

OK, you can stop when your child moves into her first apartment!

But seriously, I urge you to keep tabs on your child's pooping and peeing habits throughout the school years. This doesn't mean you need to ask your 10th-grader to describe the shape and consistency of each and every bowel movement. But occasionally asking, "Hey, how often do you use the bathroom at school?" is a wise idea.

Most kids won't volunteer that they never use the school bathroom or are having trouble pooping. When I ask my patients, their parents are often shocked to learn the kid routinely goes 8 hours without using the toilet.

Given your child's constipation history, it is particularly important to stay vigilangt throughout kindergarten and 1st grade. Compared to preschoolers, kindergarteners are expected to take a lot more responsibility for going to the restroom, but at most schools, the kindergarten bathroom is nearby. Many kids become constipated in 1st grade, when they have to take more initiative and farther. Their odds of becoming constipated skyrocket if they have teachers who believe frequent trips to the bathroom "waste" valuable class time.

Throughout grade school and beyond, periodically remind your child that laxatives, suppositories, and enemas are always available to prevent a recurrence of the difficulties the child had as a baby.

A Letter to Your Preschool

Even if your preschool has a potty-training deadline, it's worth trying to buy extra time for your child. I've written the following letter to help your case. Who knows? It just might work!

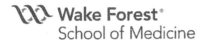
A Letter to Preschool Directors and Teachers

Dear early-childhood educator,

As the father of three young girls who attended preschool, I admire the dedication, compassion, and expertise of early childhood educators. And as a pediatric urologist, I feel compelled to offer guidance on a topic that is fraught among educators and parents: toilet training.

At my Wake Forest University clinic, I treat children of all ages who suffer from enuresis (daytime and nighttime wetting) and encopresis (stool accidents). These conditions are almost always caused by chronic constipation, a condition that often develops during toilet training but goes unnoticed by teachers and parents because the symptoms can be subtle. Even when the condition is recognized, constipation is not taken seriously enough and is vastly under-treated.

Here I'll summarize the key findings of my research and clinical practice. You can find details and studies at BedwettingAndAccidents.com, and you are welcome to contact me directly.

- **The signs of constipation are often subtle and not well known.**

Pooping frequency is not a reliable indicator of constipation! Many constipated children poop every single day. They just don't fully empty, and incomplete emptying is the root of the problem.

The telltale signs of constipation are extra-large stools and stools formed like thick logs or rabbit pellets. Other red flags: the frequent or urgent need to pee, hiding to poop, "skid marks" on underwear or diapers, recurrent urinary tract infections, stomachaches, and, most tellingly, pee or poop accidents. Pooping less than once a day is a sign of constipation, but pooping multiple times a day also can be a sign, indicating the child is not fully emptying.

It's important for preschool teachers to become familiar with these signs and alert parents so the child can receive proper treatment. Left untreated, constipation tends to worsen rather than resolve.

Children, too, are capable of learning that mushy poops are best. I recommend printing our infographic "12 Signs a Child is Constipated" for parents and posting our "How's Your Poop?" chart in your school bathrooms. Both charts are available in English and Spanish under Free Downloads on our website.

- **Accidents are never a child's fault. They are a sign that either a) the child is constipated or b) the child is not ready to toilet train.**

Accidents happen because the child's rectum, stretched by a stool pile-up, is pressing against and aggravating the bladder, causing it to "hiccup" and empty without warning. In the case of poop accidents, the stretched rectum has lost tone and sensation, so stool just drops out of the child's bottom, often without the child noticing.

None of this is within the child's control! Accidents are not a behavioral or learning issue. Suspending children from school to work on their potty skills is like suspending children with a speech delay to work on their language skills: It won't help, because these kids' issues are not related to a lack of training. They're related to a lack of treatment.

The way to resolve the accidents is to resolve the constipation, so the floppy rectum can regain its tone and sensation and stop aggravating the bladder. Even with aggressive treatment such as suppositories, enemas, and laxatives, this process can take a while. The withholding habit becomes deeply ingrained in preschool-age children, and a stretched rectum can be slow to heal. It is important to be patient as families work through these issues and to make sure children have the opportunity to use the bathroom whenever they need to, including at lunch and recess.

- **Children should not be required to complete toilet training by a certain age or date.**

I know it's easier for preschools when children are toilet trained by age 3! However, deadlines prompt many parents to train their children before they are ready, dramatically increasing the risk that the child will develop the withholding habit and become chronically constipated.

With regard to toilet training, a child's maturity is far more important than the child's age. While plenty of 2-year-olds are able to pee and poop on the toilet, many do not possess the maturity and judgment to heed their bodies' urges in a timely manner. A child's ability to use the toilet right when the urge strikes — not 20 minutes or 2 hours later — is what matters most. Many children simply do not have that kind of judgment until after their third birthday. Requiring them to do so earlier can cause lasting damage to their bladder and bowels and can cause them to end up in a clinic like mine.

Children trained before age 2 have triple the risk of developing chronic constipation and daytime wetting compared to children trained between ages 2 and 3, my research indicates.[1] However, this doesn't mean training at 2 Ð poses no risk. My research and clinical experience suggest that for most kids, it's best to wait until about age 3, and it is critical not to set deadlines!

Please do not hesitate to contact me with any questions!

Sincerely,

Steve Hodges, M.D., shodges@wakehealth.edu
Associate Professor of Pediatric Urology
Wake Forest University School of Medicine

Co-author, *Bedwetting and Accidents Aren't Your Fault*, *Jane and the Giant Poop*, and *Resolving Constipation in Babies and Toddlers: The Pre-M.O.P. Plan*

Two Potty-Training Charts

Search "potty training chart" online, and you'll find hundreds of colorful charts designed to motivate and reward children with stickers, stars, and prizes.

You won't find any charts like that here!

Our two toilet-training charts — one weekly and one monthly — are designed for parents, not children. And they have an entirely different purpose: to help you detect signs of withholding poop and pee, so you can work to nip these problems in the bud.

I'm providing two charts because some parents prefer tracking lots of detail, whereas others find details to be overwhelming.

As one mom in our support group posted:

 As one mom in our support group posted, "Now that I'm training my 4th kiddo, I know from my past mistakes that the worst thing I can do is obsess over everything detail of their toileting. It makes me stressed and in turn my kid gets stressed."

This mom paused toilet training because her daughter was demonstrating withholding behavior. (Good move!) When she resumes training, she plans to track only three indicators: 1.) spontaneous (self-initiated) poops, 2.) whether she gave her daughter an LGS, and 3.) notes.

Our 30-day potty-training chart is designed for a minimalist approach like this.

However, keep in mind that this mom also has a child on **M.O.P.** and is extremely attuned to the signs of constipation, not to mention she's toilet training her fourth child! Parents who are newer to potty training and to treating chronic constipation may benefit from taking more detailed notes, at least for a week or two.

Parents who want to monitor the process in more detail may want to use our Weekly Potty Training Chart. This chart prompts you to note how often your child pees and poops each day, along with the size and consistency of poops, treatments you are providing (laxatives and/or suppositories), and dietary and other notes.

Now, I do not recommend making yourself, or your child, nuts by logging every single trip to the toilet, the shape and consistency of every poop, every dry diaper or accident, and so on for months on end!

But even a few days of detailed tracking might help you spot trouble, which is why I've created the weekly chart. (You can download both the monthly and weekly charts from the Potty Training section of BedwettingAndAccidents.com. Samples are included in here.)

Tracking the particulars can be eye opening.

For example, you may discover a higher laxative dose is in order; a child who was pooping well on 10 ml of lactulose per day may need 20 ml during potty training.

Many parents are so focused on a child's pooping habits that they don't notice their child is going 5 or 6 hours without peeing. Others may think that because their child is pooping daily, all is fine — when, in reality, the child is just pooping a few pellets, suggesting that poop is piling up inside the rectum.

Or, you may realize that even with laxatives, your super pooper has stopped initiating poops since potty training started, and you're now using suppositories four times a week. If that's the case, I'd suggest hitting the pause button on potty training, while you treat the constipation aggressively.

I don't want to make potty training seem more complicated than it is. For children who have overcome early constipation via **PRE-M.O.P.** and who have demonstrated the signs of readiness, the process tends to go smoothly.

Still, given all you've been through, it's a good idea to keep your eye on the ball.

Weekly Potty-Training Chart

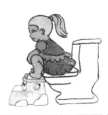

Week of: _____

MONDAY

PEEING: Total #: _____
Notes: _____

POOPING: Total #: _____
Size/consistency: _____
Notes: _____

TREATMENT NOTES
Laxative/dose: _____
LGS/enema: _____

DIETARY/OTHER NOTES
_____

TUESDAY

PEEING: Total #: _____
Notes: _____

POOPING: Total #: _____
Size/consistency: _____
Notes: _____

TREATMENT NOTES
Laxative/dose: _____
LGS/enema: _____

DIETARY/OTHER NOTES
_____

WEDNESDAY

PEEING: Total #: _____
Notes: _____

POOPING: Total #: _____
Size/consistency: _____
Notes: _____

TREATMENT NOTES
Laxative/dose: _____
LGS/enema: _____

DIETARY/OTHER NOTES
_____

THURSDAY

PEEING: Total #: _____
Notes: _____

POOPING: Total #: _____
Size/consistency: _____
Notes: _____

TREATMENT NOTES
Laxative/dose: _____
LGS/enema: _____

DIETARY/OTHER NOTES
_____

FRIDAY

PEEING: Total #: _____
Notes: _____

POOPING: Total #: _____
Size/consistency: _____
Notes: _____

TREATMENT NOTES
Laxative/dose: _____
LGS/enema: _____

DIETARY/OTHER NOTES
_____

SATURDAY

PEEING: Total #: _____
Notes: _____

POOPING: Total #: _____
Size/consistency: _____
Notes: _____

TREATMENT NOTES
Laxative/dose: _____
LGS/enema: _____

DIETARY/OTHER NOTES
_____

SUNDAY

PEEING: Total #: _____
Notes: _____

POOPING: Total #: _____
Size/consistency: _____
Notes: _____

TREATMENT NOTES
Laxative/dose: _____
LGS/enema: _____

DIETARY/OTHER NOTES
_____

Sample #1

This child pooped a "big log again," so her parent plans to increase the dose of lactulose (noted as "Need to ↑ lac").

MONDAY

PEEING: Total #: ✓✓✓✓
Notes: Mostly self-initiated; happy to pee when I reminded her.

POOPING: Total #: 1
Size/consistency: hard log again
Notes: strained a bit but proud of herself "Big poop!!!"

TREATMENT NOTES
Laxative/dose: 15 m. lac
LGS/enema: ∅

DIETARY/OTHER NOTES
drank plenty
Need to ↑ lac

Sample #2

This child took 30 ml of milk of magnesia ("MoM") plus 1 Ex-Lax square. His parent noted that Ex-Lax is helping with spontaneous pooping ("SP").

FRIDAY

PEEING: Total #: ?
Notes: Daycare said she peed "a few times"

POOPING: Total #: 2
Size/consistency: sm. rocks
Notes: 1 tiny poop @ 9 a.m.
+ snakes after dinner

TREATMENT NOTES
Laxative/dose: 30 ml MoM + 1 Ex
LGS/enema: ∅

DIETARY/OTHER NOTES
He initiated poops,
Ex-Lax helping

Potty-Training Chart
Days 1-30

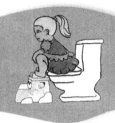

Day/Date: _____	Day/Date: _____	Day/Date: _____	Day/Date: _____	Day/Date: _____
Treatment: _____	Treatment: _____	Treatment: _____	Treatment: _____	Treatment: _____
Poops: ___ ___ ___ Total:	Poops: ___ ___ ___ Total:	Poops: ___ ___ ___ Total:	Poops: ___ ___ ___ Total:	Poops: ___ ___ ___ Total:
Poop notes: _____	Poop notes: _____	Poop notes: _____	Poop notes: _____	Poop notes: _____
Pee notes: _____	Pee notes: _____	Pee notes: _____	Pee notes: _____	Pee notes: _____
Day/Date: _____	Day/Date: _____	Day/Date: _____	Day/Date: _____	Day/Date: _____
Treatment: _____	Treatment: _____	Treatment: _____	Treatment: _____	Treatment: _____
Poops: ___ ___ ___ Total:	Poops: ___ ___ ___ Total:	Poops: ___ ___ ___ Total:	Poops: ___ ___ ___ Total:	Poops: ___ ___ ___ Total:
Poop notes: _____	Poop notes: _____	Poop notes: _____	Poop notes: _____	Poop notes: _____
Pee notes: _____	Pee notes: _____	Pee notes: _____	Pee notes: _____	Pee notes: _____
Day/Date: _____	Day/Date: _____	Day/Date: _____	Day/Date: _____	Day/Date: _____
Treatment: _____	Treatment: _____	Treatment: _____	Treatment: _____	Treatment: _____
Poops: ___ ___ ___ Total:	Poops: ___ ___ ___ Total:	Poops: ___ ___ ___ Total:	Poops: ___ ___ ___ Total:	Poops: ___ ___ ___ Total:
Poop notes: _____	Poop notes: _____	Poop notes: _____	Poop notes: _____	Poop notes: _____
Pee notes: _____	Pee notes: _____	Pee notes: _____	Pee notes: _____	Pee notes: _____
Day/Date: _____	Day/Date: _____	Day/Date: _____	Day/Date: _____	Day/Date: _____
Treatment: _____	Treatment: _____	Treatment: _____	Treatment: _____	Treatment: _____
Poops: ___ ___ ___ Total:	Poops: ___ ___ ___ Total:	Poops: ___ ___ ___ Total:	Poops: ___ ___ ___ Total:	Poops: ___ ___ ___ Total:
Poop notes: _____	Poop notes: _____	Poop notes: _____	Poop notes: _____	Poop notes: _____
Pee notes: _____	Pee notes: _____	Pee notes: _____	Pee notes: _____	Pee notes: _____
Day/Date: _____	Day/Date: _____	Day/Date: _____	Day/Date: _____	Day/Date: _____
Treatment: _____	Treatment: _____	Treatment: _____	Treatment: _____	Treatment: _____
Poops: ___ ___ ___ Total:	Poops: ___ ___ ___ Total:	Poops: ___ ___ ___ Total:	Poops: ___ ___ ___ Total:	Poops: ___ ___ ___ Total:
Poop notes: _____	Poop notes: _____	Poop notes: _____	Poop notes: _____	Poop notes: _____
Pee notes: _____	Pee notes: _____	Pee notes: _____	Pee notes: _____	Pee notes: _____
Day/Date: _____	Day/Date: _____	Day/Date: _____	Day/Date: _____	Day/Date: _____
Treatment: _____	Treatment: _____	Treatment: _____	Treatment: _____	Treatment: _____
Poops: ___ ___ ___ Total:	Poops: ___ ___ ___ Total:	Poops: ___ ___ ___ Total:	Poops: ___ ___ ___ Total:	Poops: ___ ___ ___ Total:
Poop notes: _____	Poop notes: _____	Poop notes: _____	Poop notes: _____	Poop notes: _____
Pee notes: _____	Pee notes: _____	Pee notes: _____	Pee notes: _____	Pee notes: _____

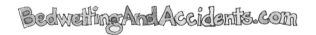

BedwettingAndAccidents.com

Sample #1

This child is taking 1 capful of Miralax daily, noted as "Mx-1 c." Her parent noted "¹/₂" a poop to denote very small poops on Thursday and Saturday. This prompted the parent to use LGS on Friday and Sunday, which improved the child's output a lot

Day/Date: Wed. 10-16	Day/Date: Thur. 10-17	Day/Date: Fri. 10-18	Day/Date: Sat. 10-19	Day/Date: Sun. 10-20
Treatment: Mx-l c	Treatment: Mx-l c	Treatment: Mx+LGS	Treatment: Mx-l c	Treatment: Mx+LGS
Poops: — — — Total: 1	Poops: ½ ⌒ — Total: ½	Poops: ✓ ✓ — Total: 2	Poops: ½ — Total: ½	Poops: — — — Total: 1
Poop notes:	Poop notes: barely – rocks	Poop notes: big pile after LGS	Poop notes: same as Thur.	Poop notes: snakes after logs
Pee notes: 😊	Pee notes: 😊	Pee notes: 😊	Pee notes: 😊	Pee notes: 😊

Sample #2

This child takes 20 or 30 ml per day of lactulose, noted as "lac." The parent increase the lactulose lose after days of meager or hard poops and saw improvement. In the "Pee notes" section, she tracked whether the child had any accidents or was dry.

Day/Date: Mon. 1-7	Day/Date: Tues. 1-8	Day/Date: Wed. 1-9	Day/Date: Thur. 1-10	Day/Date: Fri. 1-11
Treatment: lac 20	Treatment: lac 20	Treatment: lac 30	Treatment: lac 20	Treatment: lac 30
Poops: 9:30 pm Total: 2	Poops: 10 am Total: 1	Poops: — — Total: 1	Poops: — — Total: 1	Poops: 8:30 am Total: 2
Poop notes: pooped at park!	Poop notes: semi-hard	Poop notes: upped Lac-poop softer	Poop notes: log	Poop notes: more lac = better
Pee notes: plenty	Pee notes: pee accident	Pee notes: all day	Pee notes: dry	Pee notes: dry

Praise for Our Other Books

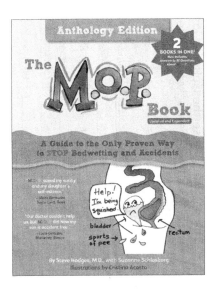

The M.O.P. Book: Anthology Edition

"It is my mission to get the word out about how incredibly effective M.O.P. is."
- Erin Wetjen, PT, specialist in pediatric incontinence Mayo Clinic, Rochester, MN

"M.O.P. saved my sanity and my daughter's self-esteem."
- Marta Bermudez, Sugar Land, TX

"M.O.P. stopped the constant accidents and allowed my child to live a normal life."
- Verified Amazon purchaser

Bedwetting and Accidents Aren't Your Fault

"Every family dealing with accidents or bedwetting should own this engaging and eye-opening book!"
- Amy McCready, founder of Positive Parenting Solutions and author of *If I Have to Tell You One More Time...*

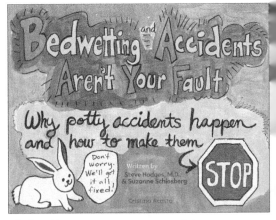

"Terrific! The illustrations are so much fun they remove any possible embarrassment, and the tone is friendly and supportive."
- Laura Markham, Ph.D., author of *Peaceful Parent, Happy Kids: How to Stop Yelling and Start Connecting*

Dr. Pooper is a ROCKSTAR!!! I'd remind my son, "What does Dr. Pooper want you to do every day?" and that would convince him to give it a try!
- Amazon verified purchaser

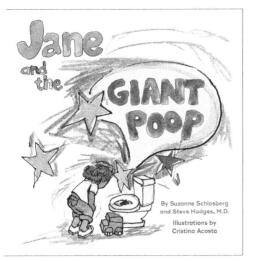

Jane and the Giant Poop

"A must-read for grown-ups, too!"
- Sally Kuzemchak, R.D., RealMomNutrition.com

"Very cute & engaging book. My kids read it 3 times first day it arrived. Helped 'normalize' their issue and bring humor to the process we are experiencing."
- Verified Amazon purchaser

"Terrific! The illustrations and humor are priceless."
- Angelique Champeau, CPNP, Director, Pediatric Continence Clinic UCSF Benioff Children's Hospital, Oakland and San Francisco

Dr. Pooper's Activity Book and Poop Calendar for Kids

"A great resource for kids with constipation and potty accidents! It helps them talk about it without embarrassment."
- Mike Garrett, M.D., Family Physician Direct MD, Austin TX

"My 5 y.o., who is following M.O.P., loves this activity book. . . He likes the mazes and 'spot the difference' pictures, and it's good for getting him talking about his potty issues.
- Verified Amazon purchaser

"I will definitely recommend this book to my patients."
- James Sander, M.D. Clinical Assistant Professor of Urology Medical University of South Carolina

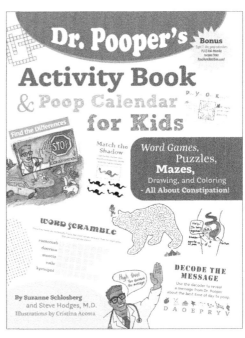

Made in the USA
Monee, IL
15 October 2024

68117855R00077